Excited,
Exhausted,
Expecting

D1396926

Excited, Exhausted, Expecting

The Emotional Life of Mothers-To-Be

Arlene Modica Matthews

A PERIGEE BOOK

A PERIGEE BOOK
Published by The Berkley Publishing Group
200 Madison Avenue
New York, NY 10016

Copyright © 1995 by Arlene Modica Matthews

Book design by Stanley S. Drate/Folio Graphics Co., Inc.

Cover illustration by Judith Leeds

First edition: March 1995

Published simultaneously in Canada.

Library of Congress Cataloging-in-Publication Data
Matthews, Arlene Modica.
    Excited, exhausted, expecting : the emotional life of mothers-to-be /
by Arlene Modica Matthews.
        p.   cm.
    "A Perigee book."
    Includes bibliographical references.
    ISBN 0-399-51885-1 (paper)
    1. Pregnancy—Psychological aspects.   I. Title.
RG560.M367   1995
618.2′4′019—dc20   94-27694
                                                                        CIP

Printed in the United States of America

10   9   8   7   6   5   4   3   2   1

For Skyler and his dad
("De Be, De Be . . . Da!")

ACKNOWLEDGMENTS

I am deeply grateful to the many women who took the time to confide their personal experiences so that this book might be of use to other expectant mothers.

Thanks to Lori Lynn Bauer, for her usual cheerful and industrious research assistance.

And to Lisa Meeks, my entry point into a network of extraordinary mothercare experts.

And to fellow psychotherapists Deborah Bershatsky, Pamela Rosenblum, Wendy Maitland, and Judith Greene for their encouragement and insightful contributions.

And to my editor, Laura Yorke, and my agent, Carla Glasser, for all their usual good works—and also for being considerate enough to become pregnant themselves while this book was being written.

Annie Fox, my pregnancy "guide" and mentor; Caralyn Shapiro, a massage therapist adept at centering both body and soul; Katie Connolly, my infectiously enthusiastic prepared childbirth instructor; and Marylou Nalducci, my wonderful, caring midwife, each helped make my own passage through pregnancy a smoother and more satisfying one than it might otherwise have been. To them I will be forever indebted.

Finally, my family and I offer our heartfelt thanks and love to the wonderful Frances Walsh. My son had the good sense to spot her while he was hanging out in heaven, waiting to be born, and cleverly arranged (along with Joe Noone's help) to make her an integral part of our lives. Without her invaluable presence, this project would never have come to fruition.

CONTENTS

INTRODUCTION

I'm Not Crazy, I'm Pregnant

*O*ften I am filled with hope; sometimes I'm consumed with dread. Often I feel blessed; sometimes I feel resentful. Sometimes I'm downright giddy. Sometimes I'm so sentimental an AT&T commercial sends me over the edge. Sometimes I feel gorgeous, earthy, and powerful. Sometimes I feel like a helium balloon with gravity shoes.

Sometimes I feel exceptionally close to my family; sometimes I wish they'd all man a space station in a galaxy far, far away. Sometimes I'd like to scream at my husband or my mother. Or that chilly receptionist in my doctor's office. Or all those casual acquaintances who keep putting their hands on my stomach. Or the virtual strangers who keep asking, "Will you breast-feed?"

Sometimes I'd just plain like to scream.

I can't decide about prenatal testing. I can't decide about natural childbirth. An abundance of advice is making me dizzy. My lack of layette is making me anxious. I can't remember where I left my "To Do" list. And hey, wait a minute—my sweater is jumping up and down! I'm being karate-chopped from the inside out. It's pretty wonderful, but also pretty . . . weird.

A delusion, you say? Certainly not. Look, I'm not crazy—I'm pregnant.

❖

These were the sorts of feelings and sensations I had in the months following my discovery that, after nearly a year of trying to conceive, I was indeed with child. And I must say, despite my years in practice as a psychotherapist—where understanding feelings was my "business"—and despite an intellectual knowledge of pregnancy's highs and lows, many of my emotions, and the depth to which I experienced them, took me by surprise.

The intensity of emotion began early in the pregnancy process for me, as it does for so many women. And it was not long after my pregnancy test's positive result that I headed off to my local bookstore with the idea of finding a volume or two to help shepherd me through the emotional maze that lay ahead. Once there, I found a plethora of books which told me, week by week, what amazing feats my fetus would be accomplishing. I also found scads of works on proper pregnancy nutrition. And if I wanted to know what to do for swollen ankles or lower back pain, I was all set. All of these books served valuable functions, but they were not going to help me contend with all the conflicting thoughts and moods which were rapidly coming to the surface.

Having come up empty-handed in my search for the appropriate book to read, I decided to write one instead. And so I spent the remaining months of my pregnancy keeping careful track of my own fluctuations of feeling, researching the state of pregnancy intently, and interviewing, individually and in group settings, nearly a hundred women from around the country who were, or recently had been, in the pregnant state.

The interview process turned out to be a thrilling experience, both from a personal standpoint (what better support network could I have devised for myself?), and a professional one. I found the vast majority of expectant mothers to be exceptionally forthcoming about their frustrations and pleasures, about their self-images, about their changing relationships with those closest to them, about the nature of their bond with their unborn children.

Though I had interviewed extensively on very personal topics for many of my previous books, I had never come across anything like the enthusiasm these women showed at being given an opportunity to share their intimate points of view and make themselves understood. In fact, in addition to the formal interviews I conducted, I was virtually deluged with pregnancy-related opinions and anecdotes at any gathering at which my project was made known. In the course of an average evening spent standing around the cheese dip at a neighbor's party, I was apt to come away with so many vivid recollections that I had to "download" my brain into my computer before going to bed.

Pregnancy is a time of profound metamorphosis on every level—on the physical level to be sure, but also on the psychological and on what one might call the "soul" levels. During its many months a woman is in a kind of altered state, between one and two, between then and thereafter. She is "open" in ways she may never quite be again. And it would be virtually impossible not to be changed by the process. Yet, incredibly, pregnancy is a much underexplored state of being.

It is my hope that this book will be one of those which will begin to fill in the glaring gap which exists in the literature of pregnancy. It is also my hope that those of you reading it will recognize some of the dilemmas you are experiencing and be able to avail yourselves of tools meant to assist you in coming to terms with them. If I've achieved my purpose here, you will learn a bit, laugh a bit, perhaps cry a bit too. And, perhaps most important, you will know that you are not alone.

To acquaint you with the structure of the book, I'll tell you that each chapter begins with a brief personal recollection of my own, reconstructed from journals kept during my nine months of pregnancy and my first three postpartum months. The balance includes perspectives of numerous other expectant mothers, as well as information gathered from a wide variety of sources, including interviews with professionals who have spent a great deal of time listening attentively to pregnant women, such as childbirth instructors, labor coaches, and midwives. At the end of each chapter, there is a section called "Privileges and Prerogatives," which contains suggestions that may help you in taking your emotional temperature and in getting your needs met.

The chapters are meant to loosely correspond chronologically with the months of the pregnancy and postpartum journey. I say *loosely,* because each chapter centers on a certain theme that some women will find themselves grappling with at an earlier or later date, depending on their temperaments and individual circumstances. I'd suggest reading the book straight through once and then returning to sections at the time they seem most relevant.

As an overview: The first chapter deals with processing the actual fact of one's pregnancy. The second discusses the sensual and perceptual shifts that pregnancy induces. The third deals with the emotional "fit" between pregnant women and their doctors or midwives. Chapter four discusses a pregnant woman's changing body image, and chapter five her evolving relationship with her baby. Chapter six focuses on the way pregnancy impacts women and their husbands. Chapter seven looks at how society chooses to "type" pregnant women and how expectant mothers feel about the roles in which they have been cast. Chapter eight discusses various sorts of late pregnancy "deadlines." Chapter nine looks at the emotional side of labor and delivery. Chapter ten is devoted to postnatal adjustments.

As you read, you will probably notice that some of the information and advice herein relates specifically to women who are pregnant for the first time. If this is a subsequent pregnancy for you, please be patient. Your "rookie" sisters often need a little extra aid and comfort. Besides, since each woman may have vastly different kinds of experiences during different pregnancies, you may well find yourself going through certain kinds of "firsts," even as a pregnancy veteran.

Of course, every expectant mother registers the realities of pregnancy in her own way. *She* gives the process its meaning, and no one should attempt to do that for her. With that in mind, please remember that this book is not meant to tell you *how* you should feel, only that you should be sure to *let yourself feel.* For your own feelings, finally, are the instruments that will help you wend your way along your particular pregnancy path while making the most of the tremendous opportunity for growth and self-knowledge which you have been given.

1 Is It True?

oh young mamas
no matter what your age is you
are born when you give birth
to a baby you start over

—ALICE OSTRIKER
The Mother-Child Papers

On a warm, damp Monday in early July, I awoke before my husband and quietly made my way into the bathroom. I fished out from the back of the cabinet beneath the sink one of those instant pregnancy answer kits whose literature promised a four-minute response to the weightiest question I had ever posed.

Was I or wasn't I? The answer kit had been lurking in the shadows for a solid year, ever since we started trying to conceive the previous summer. I'd never needed it before, but now I was ten days late, and my chest had that overripe cantaloupe feeling.

Despite this body of evidence, I was dubious. Well, dubious nothing. I was in total denial. As I paced around the living room, I tried to come up with reasons why the bright pink dot indicating pregnancy was surely not going to materialize in the window of my little white stick.

I'd been traveling a great deal in preceding weeks, on the road promoting a new book. So I told myself I was jet-lagged and "off my feed." Obviously my cycle was simply out of whack. Besides, lately, in an attempt to get really serious about this conception thing, my husband and I had tried our best to get together when our home ovulation test kits indicated conditions were optimal. This past month, though, our hectic schedules made it difficult to be so precise. Surely the universe was not so whimsical as to reward our hit-or-miss effort.

I knew my spouse, who I could hear snoring contentedly from beyond, might find it very strange if he knew just how hard I was trying to talk myself out of anticipating the very result we'd hoped for. After all, we'd become one of those mildly obsessed, googly-eyed couples that actually enjoyed sitting near babies in restaurants and on airplanes so we could triumphantly elicit a friendly grin or coo. Maybe he would have guessed I was just trying to keep myself from getting my hopes up and then being disappointed. But he would have guessed wrong.

In truth, I was busily telling myself I wasn't pregnant because I was, quite suddenly, scared witless. If the dot didn't manifest, the fear needn't be faced. So I wasn't pregnant after all, I convinced myself.

By the time my four minutes were up, I sauntered back into the bathroom prepared to flick my stick into the wastebasket and, for better or worse, resume life as I knew it. But my dot was a kind of belligerent neon magenta, and as it stared back at me it seemed to be saying, "Life as you know it is never going to resume."

The dot and I eyeballed each other for what must have been a while. Finally, I had a coherent thought, and that thought was: "I am not just me anymore. I am going to be someone's mother." And oh, it was magical and wonderful—and totally absurd.

For as I caught a glimpse of myself in the bathroom mirror, clutching the telltale white stick, looking wide-eyed and terrified, part of me—most of me—felt that, after all, I was nothing but a kid. An unprepared, ill-equipped, unworthy, and extremely uneasy 37-year-old kid. . . .

Beyond a Reasonable Doubt

For some women at certain times pregnancy comes as a genuine and total surprise. For many others, like myself, the advent of pregnancy is the culmination of a deliberate course of action meant to maximize the chances of success. In preparation for conception, coffee and alcohol may be abandoned, temperatures may be taken daily, boxer shorts may be purchased to "cool off" a husband's sperm, and prayers may be sent up petitioning the heavens for a child to care for and love. Yet even with such methodical approaches, when vague suspicions are confirmed in one manner or another and the fantasy of pregnancy becomes an actual fact, the initial reaction is often one of shock and disbelief.

In comparing notes with women about their experiences of discovering their pregnancies, it was amazing how many employed an expression like "my heart stopped" or "I couldn't catch my breath" or "the world stood still" to describe their emotional sensations upon learning of their physical states. It is as if the newly pregnant woman comprehends instantly and without question that one part of her life has been left behind forever and a new one has begun. The punctuation point between the two eras is that particular moment when the home pregnancy kit registers positive or the doctor's office calls with the momentous news. Small wonder that the punctuation mark is followed by a kind of instant backlash, with the thought, "I'm pregnant," often initially engendering its opposite thought, "No, it *can't* be true."

But, of course, it *is* true, though it may take a while to sink in. The period of astonishment may last hours, days, or even weeks, and during this time most women feel the need to reconfirm their pregnancies. One home test may lead to a second. A doctor may be asked, "Are you sure, are you *certain*?" And, even then, hours may be spent examining one's torso sideways in the mirror, looking—in vain, at this early stage—for a telltale tummy bulge.

But sooner or later, acceptance comes. The mind begins gradually to process this cataclysmic event. Now what will an expectant mother feel?

The emotions that follow the initial shock and subsequent acceptance of pregnancy vary greatly. Elation, of course, is one. Naturally many women, whether or not they planned their pregnancies, are thrilled. They may feel lucky, even blessed. And they may feel proud in the bargain, delighted to feel so undeniably female, and happily satisfied that all reproductive systems are "go." But joy is just one of a whole gamut of emotions that are common at this stage. Among those that may supplant it, or, more likely, commingle with it—for during life's rites of passage conflicting feelings so often appear in clusters—are the following:

ANXIETY

"Before I got pregnant," recalled Melissa, who conceived her daughter at age 32, "all I could think of were images of the Gerber baby ads. I couldn't wait to get one of those precious, adorable bundles for myself. When I found out I was really going to have a baby, I was suddenly horrified that I had no control over my life. This will change everything, I thought, disrupt everything—my career, my marriage. I was so alarmed that I couldn't conjure up that Gerber baby picture any longer. All I could visualize was an inconsolable, crying infant, just waiting to blow my well-organized life to smithereens."

SELF-DOUBT

"Because I myself am a teacher," remembered Susan, who bore the first of her two sons at 26, "I had the notion that I would make a naturally good mother. Better than most, I assumed. How smug I was, watching other women at their wits' end, chasing their out-of-control kids all over the supermarket, thinking, 'Oh, I'll never be like that.' But when I became pregnant with Tommy I had an instant sense of inadequacy. I felt I didn't know anything at all, especially about infants. I was a *fraud*. I'd never be able to pull this off."

FEAR

"For me," said Jacqueline, whose twins were conceived when she was 34, "mixed in with excitement was fear of the physical aspects of what I would be going through. Childbirth? Forget it! I'd seen all those TV shows and movies with some poor woman writhing in a hospital bed and everyone around her hollering, 'Push, push,' at the top of their lungs. Even though I definitely wanted to be a mother, I kept thinking, 'How am I going to get out of this labor and delivery part?' "

EMBARRASSMENT

"This may sound silly," confessed Elyssa, who had her daughter when she was 28 years old, "but although I was glad, I could practically feel myself blushing every time I thought about the fact that I'd gotten pregnant. In fact, right away, I had a memory come up from my childhood. I was a little kid, maybe five or six, and I overheard my grandmother tell my parents that one of my older cousins was pregnant. This seemed to cause a lot of talk and get a big reaction. Years later, I found out it was because she was not married and 'in trouble,' as the saying went back then. But as a little girl, all I knew was that this 'pregnant' thing seemed to command a lot of attention. So later I climbed on my dad's lap and said, 'I'm pregnant too.' Both my parents turned white as sheets and my mother yelled, 'Oh, God forbid it should happen to you.' Well, for some reason this always stuck in my mind.

"Now, after all these years, it was like I had done something I wasn't supposed to do, even though I was married. And now I'd have to tell everyone, even my *parents*. I dreaded the time when I would start to show and then get really big and, well, funny-looking. Because then everybody would know, you know, that I'd gone and done this thing. You know, *sex*!"

ENTRAPMENT

"Even though mine was a planned pregnancy," said Jacqueline, who conceived soon after going off the pill at age 30, "I kept thinking, 'Wait a minute, let me go back and mull this over a little more.' But that was impossible. There simply was no going back. My husband was ecstatic. And we'd told everyone we were going to try to get pregnant that year. And sure I wanted to be a mother, someday. But now? Was this really a good idea?

Of course, all this was academic. It was too late for second guessing. For the first time in my life I had done something that couldn't be undone. Well, I suppose technically it could have been undone, but that was unthinkable. So why was I thinking it, even for a split second? Oh, that made me feel really selfish. Now I felt really trapped, because I thought I shouldn't even share my thoughts with anyone."

SADNESS
"After the initial shock came a quick burst of triumph and relief, but then for the next few weeks, there was a deep sense of sorrow," recalled Marilyn, who became pregnant at 42 after two tries at in vitro fertilization. "Even now it's hard to describe exactly, but it was almost as if I was in mourning. The gloomy feelings overwhelmed and confounded me. For years, my husband and I had been brokenhearted because we couldn't have kids. Now a miracle had occurred, and I was saturated with grief. Why, I couldn't say. Everyone told me it was 'just hormones,' but I found that hard to swallow. It felt like it came from my soul, not just from my glands."

These recollections represent a wide range of thoughts and emotions, and the women quoted may appear to have had very different states of mind. But they do have one important thing in common. They never *expected* to have the feelings they had with relation to their pregnancies. What they imagined they would experience was unadulterated bliss. What they got, at best, was a mixed bag. Their unanticipated misgivings felt incongruous to them. Why, they wondered, did their feelings not fit the situation?

Not too surprisingly, such musing led to yet another feeling . . .

Welcome to Maternal Guilt

Self-recrimination is often the result when people greet an event the culture has deemed pleasurable with emotions that tend to be categorized as unpleasant, such as anxiety, sadness, or fear. When it comes to pregnancy in particular the cultural message we as women are given over and over again is that discovering one is with child is an occasion for rejoicing, as indeed it often is.

But each and every other feeling mentioned above is equally as valid, and should be equally honored as an important part of the psychic journey that pregnancy mandates. Indeed, when you think about it, why *shouldn't* pregnancy generate an emotional upheaval? That seems very reasonable considering the magnitude of what is happening.

Are you anxious? That's appropriate. The act of ushering a new life into this world will require you to reinvent every aspect of your private world. Throughout your entire pregnancy one of the things you will hear people say over and over to you is that "your whole life will change." Annoying as this maxim may seem, it is true. In many ways it will change for the better, but in order for this to be so, you will have to relinquish many of the things you now take for granted.

If this is your first child, you will have to forfeit the freedom to come and go as you please, without concern for feedings and nap times and baby bag toting and diaper changing etiquette. You will have to relinquish one sort of relationship with your spouse—one with which you have probably grown quite comfortable—and forge another, more complicated bond. Even if you already have children, you will have to reorganize everything once again, both on physical and psychological planes, making room not only in your home but in your heart for another. Given all this, only someone with the self-awareness of a Rice Krispy would be able to forego anxiety entirely.

Do you doubt your ability to handle the formidable tasks before you? That's only natural. Motherhood is a series of never ending challenges. Just when one ends, six or seven more take its place. And this will seem to happen on a weekly basis for more or less the rest of your life. That's enough to humble anyone with sense enough to think about it.

Are you frightened by thoughts of labor and childbirth? If you've never been through it, the idea of actually getting a baby out from inside your body is virtually incomprehensible, rather like getting a ship out of a bottle. Sure, on an intellectual level, you know women give birth every day, and have for millennia. But does that really help you process the notion that *you're* going to have to do it? Probably not.

In our society, supposedly so sophisticated and "liberated," we are taught very little about the physical process of childbirth. We are told little about how to prepare our bodies and less still about how to prepare our minds. What's more, for reasons that will be discussed later on, the mothers of women who are of childbearing age today have, for the most part, handed down a legacy of negative messages about birthgiving. Understandably, fear is par for the pregnancy course.

What about embarrassment? Is it normal to have such a "silly" feeling at this time? Again, let's look at the cultural context. At one point, pregnancy was referred to as "confinement," and women were literally sequestered from the time they began to show until the time they gave birth. Of course that time is past. Just as is the time—not so very long ago—that it was impermissible to say the word "pregnant" on television. But residues of such arcane attitudes remain, as language attests. Even today, the Spanish word for pregnancy is *embarazo*—literally, embarrassment.

As teenage girls in "hygiene" classes, most of us were taught how not to get pregnant, which is all fine and well considering the potentially devastating consequences of ignoring such information. However, we were never taught how to *be* pregnant, and comfortable with it, when the suitable time in our lives arrived. Deep down, the command "Thou shalt not get pregnant" seems to linger in the minds of many. To defy it, some feel, is to call attention to oneself as slightly "naughty."

What's more, though we may not like to admit it, even to ourselves, we may think that to be pregnant is to look somehow "funny." Even if this is not how *we* view pregnancy personally, we are afraid that this is how it may be viewed by others. And even if we do not fear others will perceive us as somehow unattractive during our childbearing months, we may be made uneasy by the certainty that others will, in any case, be inspecting us with heightened attentiveness.

What about feelings of entrapment? Those too can be utterly appropriate. Once having elected to bear a child, one finds the process relentless, to say the least. Month after month, one's body waxes larger. After a point, the baby grows more and more active, more "present" with each passing week. Every mirror, every stretched-out waistband, every kick and nudge serves to remind an expectant mother of her circumstance and of the enormity of her commitment. It is entirely appropriate to feel, at least from time to time, that your life and your body are no longer your own. They're not.

Lastly, what about sadness? Your life is about to be enhanced in so many ways, and you keep reminding yourself that a great many women might give anything to trade places with you. But you must remind yourself too that all gain involves loss and all loss involves mourning. Do you have a right to be sad? Why not? You have a right to mourn your existence as it is, for it will never be that way again.

All in all, you have a right to think and feel *anything* as you move forward toward your revised life. In all my personal and professional experience, I have never met an expectant mother who has sustained only feelings of joy and delight, to the exclusion of all else, during the nine months of her pregnancy. Yet I have encountered many a woman who does not like to *admit* that she feels anything else.

Such a woman may assume what I call the Pollyanna Pregnant attitude. She tells others only how happy she is, just as she tries to convince herself of the same. If she feels a disquieting undertow tugging at her professed bliss, she tries as hard as she can to press it down deeper and deeper, until it's so effectively buried that she can almost will herself to forget it's there. Yet it remains there, still.

And if not given its due, this undertow may assert itself at some point to disrupt her equanimity much more than if she'd allowed herself to deal with it in the first place. At some point, it may manifest itself in stress-related physical symptoms (such as back pain, headaches, and the like), in impulsive emotional outbursts (perhaps leading to draining, redundant quarrels with those she loves most), in poor decision-making, and in a diminished ability to take good care of herself and her unborn charge.

It is common for expectant mothers to believe that having complex and conflicting feelings about their pregnancies makes them somehow "bad." But it does not. It simply makes them human.

It is also common to fear that if they allow any doubts to enter their minds that they will be "punished." They may dread that the unthinkable will happen and that they may cause harm to their babies if they let themselves feel anxious, frightened, or angry, or if, for instance, they fleetingly entertain a thought such as "I wish this pregnancy had come at a more convenient time." (A very common thought, there being no truly convenient time to rearrange one's entire life.)

But no baby has ever been poorly affected by having a mother who was kind and nurturing to herself during her pregnancy. Quite the contrary. And part of that self-nurturing involves giving yourself permission to feel whatever it is you feel without chastising yourself.

Hormones: A Hostile Takeover?

Before going any further with the subject of reactions to pregnancy, this is probably a good time to address one of the questions that you may already be asking yourself with regards to your shifting moods. Often, when an expectant mother feels an unexpected emotion she is prone to wonder: Is it me or my hormones?

As everyone knows, from the instant conception takes place there is a massive hormonal shift in a woman's body, emanating from her own glands and from the developing placenta, that produces all manner of miraculous events.

It's true that these hormonal changes can have not only a physiological but a psychological impact. At this point it's unthinkable that anyone who studies either the mind or the body would seriously dispute their interrelationship. Our emotional state is doubtless affected by our body chemistry. But the reverse is also true. This makes for a complicated chicken-and-egg dynamic that we don't yet, and may never, fully understand. It also makes it a gross oversimplification to attribute our emotions solely to hormonal influences.

While the presence of certain hormones at certain levels can undoubtedly *intensify* emotions, it would be foolhardy to conclude that a hormone, in and of itself, is manufacturing emotions from out of the blue. Psychological and social factors should never be discounted as potential powerful codeterminants of one's emotional state.

In Greek, the root *hormon* means "to excite." And this is often exactly what hormones seem to do with regard to emotions. So rather than thinking of your pregnancy-related hormones as invidious substances which are going to transform you from a placid Jekyll to an out-of-control Hyde, it's more realistic to think of them as psycho-physiological "spices." In cooking, of course, spices change the potency of a dish but do not alter its basic ingredients.

If you are feeling stressed or blue with regards to your pregnancy, chances are there are *plenty* of reasons to feel the way you do. But certainly, if the levels of stress or depression are so intense they feel out of character for you, consider that in addition to the fact that your psyche is attempting to cope with a challenging and perhaps altogether new situation, it could also well be that your feelings are being "spiced" by hormones. Take that for what it's worth. A part of the picture—no less, but no more.

It is tempting indeed to chalk up all of one's initial emotional reactions to pregnancy (not to mention the emotional ups and downs that may well come later in the process) to a case of hormonal shenanigans. Tempting because this gets one off the hook with regards to owning, and owning up to, all one's feelings (especially the ones we tend to brand as negative and from which we'd like to disassociate ourselves).

But one would be wise to avoid this rationale. To blame all your emotional ups, downs, and in-betweens *strictly* on hormonal antics is to do yourself a disservice. Such an attitude can make you experience yourself as simply "along for the ride" of pregnancy, a vulnerable victim of a hostile takeover in your body. It can cut you off from your basic instincts. This is never a good idea, and especially not now, for as we'll see one's instincts are especially keen in the pregnant state.

Also, if you attribute all your reactions and moods to hormonal causes, your tendency may be to keep silent about your emotions. Even if you do occasionally admit to a bad mood or nagging fear, you will be likely to quickly hush up again once anyone else reminds you that it's "only your hormones" talking. You will likely compound any difficult feelings you may have by keeping a tight lid on them, and you will not be doing anyone any good by letting yourself be wiped out by others' dismissive and condescending remarks.

Last of all, if you see every problem as a nail, the only tool you'll ever use will be a hammer. In other words, if you think every pregnancy-related emotion is hormone-generated, you may assume they should all be treated in the same fashion and try to pound them down out of conscious awareness. In your "hammering" mode, you will never take the time to consider what it is that might actually make you feel better—be it a proverbial shoulder to cry on, a tension-relieving back rub, an hour to yourself, or an emphatic hug—and to ask for it.

Your hormonal structure is a complex and valuable part of what makes you you. It's wise not to disregard it, but it ought not be focused on to the exclusion of other parts, such as psyche and spirit. For to disown any part of you is to undermine your entire self. And just now is when your "self" must stand solid and strong.

For you have work to do, not the least of which is spreading the word of your pregnancy. Now you not only have to deal with your reactions, but with the reactions of your family, friends, and colleagues as well.

We're Pregnant

In nearly every instance, of course, the first person informed that a woman is a mother-to-be is the baby's father-to-be. Indeed, sharing the news with one's partner is such a major milestone in the journey of pregnancy that numerous situation comedies have mined this rich emotional territory. In the world of television, the plot generally goes: Woman learns of her pregnancy, becomes instantly overjoyed and plans a romantic interlude during which she will surprise her husband with her bulletin. The interlude (which, naturally, includes some hilarious and obligatory sitcom mix-ups and misunderstandings) culminates in her husband's becoming equally overjoyed—and then fainting dead away.

In reality, most newly expectant mothers have too much on their minds to contrive a romantic tête-à-tête, and instead tend to track down their husbands wherever they may be and blurt out, "I'm pregnant," or very likely, "*We're* pregnant" with little or no prelude. These days, thanks again to the advent of home pregnancy testing kits, a man often learns of his wife's condition only moments after she learns of it. And often both are faced with trying to process their own complicated reactions while attempting simultaneously to read the other's deepest feelings. Thus begins the complex emotional *pas de deux* that will continue for the next nine months between mates as they try their new and shifting roles on for size.

What is typically a husband's first reaction to pregnancy? Like women's responses, men's run the gamut. Many fathers-to-be are ebullient, of course. But many are incredulous as well.

"I remember calling my husband in from the backyard and waving a stick at him frantically," recalled Eve. "I kept yelling, 'It's blue. It's blue. The stick is blue.' We had only just begun trying to have a baby and here it was. I was beside myself, I just couldn't believe it was true. Not so soon! It couldn't possibly be. My husband, who had never seen a home pregnancy test and didn't know what in the world this stick signified, looked at me like I'd lost my marbles. When he finally understood, he still didn't believe it. He was in total denial the entire weekend. Until I got to a doctor on Monday, he wouldn't believe there wasn't some mistake."

Naturally, men's reactions to their wives' pregnancies also include various misgivings and fears. Some of their anxieties are identical to women's, and involve concerns about the impending loss of freedom and the looming responsibilities of parenthood. This can be the case even if the couple has already had other children.

"When I announced my third pregnancy," said 31-year-old Julie, "my husband's immediate response was to let out a whoop. But then he held me tight and said, 'Oh oh, *what have we done?* Now the kids will outnumber us. How are we going to pull this off?' I could tell he was excited, but also really scared, like me."

Not surprisingly, some women recalled their husbands' first fears were financial ones. For money is like a blank screen onto which it is easy to project several overlapping anxieties:

"After what seemed like a minute of silence, my husband went into a money panic," said 27-year-old Louise, who happily announced her first pregnancy by telephone as her husband, a motion picture cameraman, was away on a film location. "He said he was afraid he'd never work again, that he couldn't imagine where we would live, that he could never take care of us all, that we'd never find a solution. He seemed so childish himself, when I could only think of the good times I'd have with our child-to-be. I couldn't stand it."

Whatever a husband's response is, it will give his wife more grist for her already churning emotional mill. Sometimes it will calm her down, reassure her. Sometimes it will upset her. Interestingly enough, the deciding factor as to whether a woman feels positively or negatively about her husband's response to her news is often not what emotions he evidences but whether or not those emotions resonate with hers, and therefore seem to validate her feelings.

For example, Eve and Julie said they had no problem with their husbands' responses because those responses mirrored some of their own doubts. True, Eve's husband was in denial, but in a way so was she. Neither was prepared to assimilate quickly the fact that they had conceived on their very first attempt. Julie too felt in sync with her husband when he professed his overwhelmed state. Like him, she was also wondering how they could fit a third child into their already full lives and complicated household, and when her husband held her tight she had the sense that they were truly "in it together."

Louise, as is obvious from her remarks, was less than pleased with her husband's panicked reaction. Largely caught up in pleasant anticipation, she did not appreciate being brought down by anything so sobering as fiscal concerns. Nor did she care for her husband's initial frenzied approach, which she perceived as immature. Most likely if she herself had been experiencing financial fears at the time she would not have deemed his reaction so inappropriate. But, for the moment anyhow, she was unperturbed by such matters and became riled that they loomed so predominant for her partner.

Intriguingly, resonance between their husbands' reactions and their own is so important to some women that even if their spouses are completely exhilarated at the prospect of a baby in the house, women may not relish their husbands' responses if they themselves are not feeling in a totally exhilarated state at this early juncture.

"After taking not one but two different pregnancy tests, to be certain, I marched out of the bathroom in a daze," remembered 36-year-old Annalee. "I was suddenly so scared of so many things I just wanted to cry. My husband Bob started shouting and jumping up and down. He wanted to tell the whole world, and was oblivious to my long face. The more euphoric he got, the more traumatized and guilty I felt. When he finally noticed I was pale and biting my lower lip, he said, 'I thought this was what you wanted. Well, at least one of us is happy.' Then I really burst into tears."

Had Bob been a little more observant at the start and taken a more restrained approach, Annalee might have been better able to cope with her worries and felt freer to unburden herself to her spouse. Though there is no blame to be placed on Bob, who was simply being, as his wife put it, "his usual exuberant self," his enthusiasm was not what she wanted to hear at that particular moment. Only when he later apologized did his wife begin to feel he understood her.

The husband/wife relationship will undergo many changes

as a pregnancy proceeds, and more still when a brand-new, totally reliant, tiny baby finally arrives to turn the family dynamic
inside out and upside down. In the course of this book, there will
be more to say about the impact of pregnancy and childbirth on
a marriage. At this point, however, suffice it to say that if newly
pregnant women everywhere could ask for one thing from their
husbands, it would probably be simply: *Understand me, or at
least do your best to try.* It is a request so simple, yet, as we'll
see, sometimes so difficult to grant, as husbands grapple with
their own very real and very urgent issues regarding the challenges that lie ahead.

But for now, let's leave the subject of husbands for one
equally as charged emotionally. For just as there is one key thing
a pregnant woman wants from her spouse at this critical time in
her life, there is something else she wants from another loved
one that is equally significant.

Telling Mother You'll Be a Mother

Phyllis Chesler has written that for a woman to become a
mother is to honor the woman that gave birth to her. And it is
easy to see how this is so. To take on the task of mothering is to
validate it, and by embracing this new role a woman is, in fact,
communicating to her own mother on some profound, primal
level that she wishes, regardless of their differences (myriad
though they may be) to join ranks with her. It is a message one
hopes will be well received, and in return for dispatching it, a
pregnant woman generally longs for one thing. It is the very
same thing she has most likely wanted from her mother all her
life: Approval.

For most of us, regardless of how independent we like to
think we are, a major goal of our lives from infancy through
childhood through adolescence and on into adulthood is to win
Mother's praise and encouragement and to secure her blessing
on our endeavors. Whether or not our relationship with Mother
is rocky, she is, after all, the woman who nurtured us, the first

female with whom we identified, and the first we longed to emulate.

Most of us did emulate Mother when we tried on her high heels, or tied her apron around us, or splashed on her perfume. Some of us even followed in her footsteps by choosing a particular kind of man to marry, or a particular school or career path. For the vast majority of women, each of these junctures was far more satisfying when Mother bestowed her benediction. But now, as an expectant mother herself, a daughter is going for the big one—the ultimate rite of passage that says I too am now a full participant of the community of women. I too am privy to the secrets, to the power.

Alas, for some, attaining Mother's blessing for any of our rites of passage, including this paramount one, is as frustrating as seeking the elusive Holy Grail. Mother/daughter relationships are a complex business, and though a deep, abiding love is at the core of nearly all of them, that does not seem to prohibit many a mother from offering up a less than ideal response to a daughter's announcement of pregnancy. Indeed, many newly pregnant women find they work up quite a case of nerves getting ready to let their mothers in on their little secret. They fear that any problematical dynamic that has existed in their relationship may be rekindled at this highly sensitive moment. Often they are right.

If your relationship with your mother has always been marked by competitive striving, you may get a less desirable reaction than you'd hoped. For example:

"That's wonderful, dear, but don't gain too much weight. Those doctors today have you girls eat like whales, and you know you already have a hearty appetite. *I* only gained fifteen pounds when I was carrying you—and I dropped it the week after delivery."

Similarly, if your perennially worried mother has always felt the need to control you, lest you do something reckless, you may hear a refrain that typifies her attitude:

"Oh my gosh, you'd better get off your feet. Let me get you a drink of water. You have to keep hydrated, you know. So, when are you going to have the tests that tell you if everything's OK? You *are* going to have all the tests, aren't you?"

If your mother is prone to a blurring of boundaries, periodically forgetting that you and she are no longer umbilically attached, she may seem confused as to just *who* it is that's pregnant anyway, rhapsodizing:

"Oh, how wonderful, darling. We're having a baby. I've always wanted another baby. I can't wait to tell my friends I'm going to be a mother. Oops, I mean grandmother."

Needless to say, such responses may provoke feelings of keen disappointment in a pregnant daughter. Here you may have been expecting your condition to smooth over the rough patches in your mother/daughter bond, only to find that your areas of conflict are being underscored. It is tempting to throw up one's hands in defeat. But at the same time, the intense drive within you to please your mother and to have her appreciate you is likely to keep your quest for the Grail alive.

Over the course of a pregnancy, the relationship you have with your mother, like that you have with your husband, will take on new dimensions. Where your mother is concerned, you may seek to identify yourself with her in certain ways, and disassociate yourself in others (assuring yourself, "I'll never make this or that mistake with my child"). And over the next nine months, even if your mother herself does not change, it is likely that your perceptions of her will.

But much of that still lies ahead. For now, you will need to handle your mother's initial reflex to the event of your pregnancy. If you have already weathered a less than ideal response from your mother, it may lessen the hurt to know that she is likely acting out of her own anxieties about your well-being as well as any unresolved conflicts she may have about childbearing. If, on the other hand, you have not yet informed your mother and have trepidations about doing so, you may want to keep in mind the strategy of a woman who managed to anticipate her mother's reaction to her pregnancy and then head it off at the pass:

"My mother usually gets so worried about me that I end up taking care of her," said Ellen, who became pregnant for the first time at 39 years of age. "This time, I did not want that to happen. I felt strongly that I wanted to be taken care of, that I deserved it. So I instructed her as to what to do. I called her up and said, 'Mom, I've got some big news and I want you to be really happy for me.' I also told her that if she felt anxious about my pregnancy that she should talk to my sister about it."

According to Ellen, this strategy worked beautifully, and I heartily join her in recommending it. Not only can asking for what you want from your mother spare you a lot of Sturm und Drang at this sensitive moment, it can also pave the way for making some of the changes that may be necessary as your relationship with her begins, inevitably, to be redefined.

Going Public

Once they have told their inner circle of husband and immediate family what is happening, pregnant women are faced with the conundrums of deciding who else to tell in what order, and of dealing with the various and sundry reactions of friends and colleagues.

Just how to go public with one's pregnancy can be a very delicate matter. It often requires diplomacy, for just about everyone wants to be high on your list of confidantes and many are insulted if word "leaks" to them before you've contacted them personally. In some instances, it also may require a substantial degree of tact, for there may be friends who have tried unsuccessfully to conceive and who may be hard pressed to summon up the hearty sort of congratulations with which others are showering you.

Finally, disclosing one's pregnancy at work may require a healthy dose of public relations skill. Even genuinely supportive bosses and coworkers may find it difficult to conceal their uneasiness about how pregnancy and motherhood will affect a woman's job performance, not to mention whether or not she will be continuing on the job at all once the baby arrives. No matter how many assurances she provides to the contrary, some may be dubious about her long-term commitment to her career.

There is simply no telling exactly what reactions a woman will provoke as she takes her pregnancy public. With luck, most people will offer appropriate, if not perfect, responses. But one might do well to decide in advance not to be felled by any inappropriate replies to the news, such as the friend who responds, "Well, it's nice to know *someone* who's fertile," or the coworker who wants to know, "Can I have your office while you're on maternity leave?"

It would be wonderful indeed if everyone who impacts on your life could show acute sensitivity to your needs. Alas, not everyone may want you to have all your feelings concerning your pregnancy. They may want you to have *their* feelings instead. It is, however, not incumbent upon you to cooperate with them.

Should you feel yourself tempted to do so, *or to do anything else that will undermine your processing the news of your pregnancy in the way that makes the most sense for you personally,* you may want to consult the following list of Privileges and Prerogatives. It is the first of ten such compendiums that are meant to serve as handy reminders to see you through the nine months of pregnancy and the postpartum period.

❖ AN EXPECTANT MOTHER'S PRIVILEGES
AND PREROGATIVES

You have the right to remain silent. In eighteenth- and nineteenth-century France the official herald of pregnancy was an owl. According to popular belief, if the winged creature perched on a rooftop and hooted, the lady of the house below was said to be with child.[1] Lacking such fine feathered gossips here and now, it is up to each woman to choose who she wants to tell she is pregnant, and when she wants to tell them. Once you have informed anyone whose participation in the process you consider essential from the start (for example, your spouse), do not feel pressured to clue anyone else in unless you feel ready. Parents, siblings, in-laws, friends, and colleagues can *all* wait until you have had some time to process things for yourself.

Nothing you say—or think or feel—should be held against you. If you find yourself having unanticipated emotions at this time, and if some of those emotions seem to conflict with each other, do not consider yourself less "worthy" of motherhood than you'd hoped. Instead, show yourself some compassion.

Given the magnitude of your discovery, you have the right—yes, even the obligation—to let yourself experience the many nuances of your feelings. You are entitled to speak aloud about your emotions if you wish (choose an ear you know to be sympathetic for the greatest benefit), but if you do not wish to share all your beliefs and attitudes at this juncture, consider keeping a journal in which to record them. Often giving verbal or written shape to a thought or feeling renders it far less intimidating and troubling.

Get a temporary restraining order. You have the right to instruct your relatives and friends as to the nature of the response you wish to elicit. If there is anyone in your personal life whose response you are dreading (even if it is very well meant, such as a nervous mother's lament), try prefacing your announcement with a very specific guideline such as "I want to tell you something that I know will make you very glad. And I can't wait to hear how glad you are." Even if their full cooperation is not forthcoming, at the very least you will begin to get in the habit of defining and requesting what it is you want. At best, you could establish a very healthy precedent that will serve you well throughout your pregnancy.

Look at the big picture. It cannot be said often enough that while hormones play a key role in the process of pregnancy, we are not merely a compendium of chemicals. From the holistic point of view that is today the vanguard of research in fields as diverse as medicine and immunology, psychology and philosophy, we are all interacting systems of body and mind. Both are now working together to nurture the baby inside you. To give short shrift to any aspect of this mind/body unity is to deprive yourself of vital resources you will need for negotiating your pregnancy and postpartum months.

Finally, and above all:

Give yourself permission to change and keep on changing. It is a testament to Mother Nature's good sense that pregnancy takes nine months to unfold. During these months, you will undoubtedly become reacquainted with yourself on a regular basis. Pregnancy as metamorphosis is a fact of life, and a necessary one, considering how much additional change this new child will bring to your life after it is born.

Hence, you are about to learn things about your priorities, your relationships, your dreams and your demons, your fortes and foibles, your values and your expectations that you never realized before. And just when you think you've settled into a groove, you will surprise yourself, and those around you, once more. Get used to it. And stay mindful always of this crucial dynamic of change.

For even now, as your second month of pregnancy dawns, your senses and sensibilities are beginning to shift in new, amazing, and sometimes confounding ways.

2 Shifting Senses

We live on the leash of our senses . . . We like to think
we are finely evolved creatures, in . . . pantyhose and
chemise, who live many millennia and mental de-
tours away from the cave, but that's not something
our bodies are convinced of.

—DIANE ACKERMAN
A Natural History of the Senses

*By the time I was six or seven weeks pregnant I could smell
everything, and I mean everything, with the acuity of a blood-
hound. Someone cooking lasagna three floors up? I could tell
you precisely how much oregano was in the sauce. Someone
sporting a dab of new cologne sprinkled on twelve hours ago?
I could tell the instant they entered the room that their aroma
had been altered.*

*This newfound olfactory ability might have made for an
interesting, perhaps even rather pleasant, phenomenon if I
lived in, say, the desert Southwest near a growth of sagebrush.
But I lived in Manhattan—land of taxicab exhaust, restaurant dumpsters, Central Park Port-O-Sans. To make matters
worse it was August, when everything is especially pungent.
The assault on my nasal receptor cells was overwhelming and
left me feeling besieged, beleaguered, and more than a little
short-tempered.*

*I pored over my pregnancy texts to try and discover why
this was happening to me. But it was not entirely clear what*

was accountable. I suppose that from an evolutionary stand-point it all makes sense. Back in the primal forest of human-kind's dawn, a pregnant Homo sapiens probably enjoyed a much better chance of carrying her baby to term if she could sniff out available food sources, not to mention dangerous predators, with greater accuracy. When it came to noses, the Darwinian rule may well have been "the survival of the sharpest."

But in my urban environment, I felt a new vulnerability. And indeed, smell was not the only reason why. Suddenly, all my senses seemed more, well, hypersensitive. I saw and heard things I'd never noticed before. My stimulus barriers, so es-sential to daily life in a hectic metropolis, seemed to be eroding.

Even at home, far from the madding crowd, I experienced a sort of sensory overload. The texture of my clothes against my skin felt different depending on how they'd been laun-dered. I reacted more strongly than ever to different sorts of music, to various colors, and even to the differing tempera-ments of the people around me.

As for taste, well that was a whole new ball game, with former favorite foods now tasting foul and cravings develop-ing for items of which I'd always steered clear. Kale and col-lard greens seemed strangely appealing, while I could not have stared down an egg-over-easy for any extravagant re-ward, nor even have begun to imagine how any sane person could have anything to do with a yellow pepper.

All in all, one thing was clear. My "altered state" had re-arranged all my perceptions, and the psychological impact of that was both intriguing and unnerving. . . .

Pickles and Ice Cream

When it comes to an expectant mother's shifting perceptions, desires, and dislikes there is, in the popular consciousness, per-haps no association so commonly made as that of pregnancy with food cravings and aversions. In fact it sometimes seems the newly pregnant couple can hardly go anywhere without the husband being ribbed about his wife's newfound devotion to the clichéd combo of pickles and ice cream.

Obviously, not every pregnant woman experiences a yen for pickles and ice cream per se, but chances are nearly every one will hanker for some food or other, sometimes one they had little or no interest in before the pregnancy began. At the same time they'll develop aversions to other foods, perhaps ones that were much relished at an earlier time. Heightened interest in some foods with auxiliary disdain for others (usually starting at about the second month of pregnancy, but sometimes even sooner) is just one aspect of the many ways in which a pregnant woman's senses alter and adjust. But it exemplifies some fundamental and important points about these permutations that every expectant mother ought to know.

As each shift in the sense comes about, one is likely to feel a bit bewildered. It's natural to wonder why this or that taste or smell or other sensation is more palatable, or more offensive, than it previously was. Is this a strictly chemical phenomenon, or could there be more involved as well? Are the changes mandated by the developing baby or by her own being?

Heightened estrogen and heightened senses do tend to correlate in pregnancy, as they do in the first half of a woman's menstrual cycle. However, many pregnancy-related phenomena seem to dovetail, and their aspects appear to be engendered by numerous overlapping causes.

Let's take our proverbial pickles and ice cream as an example. Suppose at some point in her pregnancy a woman literally awakens at 3 A.M. with an urgent yearning for these particular edibles—a longing so powerful that she does, in fact, arouse her slumbering spouse. Where might such a longing be coming from, and what might it signify?

Theories abound.

From a physiological standpoint: The pickles are high in salt content. And since increased blood volume during pregnancy lowers the sodium levels of a mother-to-be, it is harder for her to experience saltiness as a taste. Hence, she wants more of it.

From a neurobiological standpoint: The ice cream, a sweet,

stimulates the production of serotonin, a neurotransmitter of calm which will serve a woman well during the rigors of pregnancy and the coming arduous demands of childbirth.

From a psychological standpoint: A request of this nature made of one's husband could be a test the woman is administering (albeit unconsciously or semiconsciously) to have the husband prove how committed he is to her and how participatory he wishes to be in the pregnancy process. If he actually attempts, even unsuccessfully, to procure her unorthodox snack in the wee hours of the morning, he passes muster.

From a more incorporeal standpoint: It is the baby that wants pickles and ice cream, or the substances they contain, for its own purposes, and the mother is simply acting as its agent. So unified are mother and child that the mother automatically does the baby's culinary bidding.

Each hypothesis contains a kind of logic.

It's hard to deny that there is a nutritional element to many cravings. Pregnant women whose diets have been too low in calcium and other minerals have been known to crave and consume clay (in the southern United States) and even termite mounds (in parts of Africa).[1] It's not hard to view my own yen for kale as a similar example of heeding the body's ineluctable wisdom, for greens contain the folic acid necessary for the growth of a healthy baby.

It seems reasonable too that a pregnant woman would be driven toward foods that increase production of natural relaxants and painkillers. A potent incentive for the staunch vegetarians who frequently find themselves heading for the nearest greasy spoon during pregnancy is that grease-laden foods, alas, help generate endorphins.

But it's equally valid to say that a craving may signify an underlying emotional dynamic, such as a woman's need to enlist her husband's nurturance. Any particular craving may, in any number of ways, relate to an expectant mother's powerful need to be comforted. Thus, she might turn to the foods that she associated with her own childhood and her own mother (mashed potatoes and tapioca, anyone?) or to any food that she regularly consumed during a period of her life that is especially meaningful to her. As one woman recalled:

> "For week after week during my pregnancy, all I could think of at lunchtime was this particular tuna fish sandwich I used to get years before at a certain deli.
>
> "I now worked across town from this deli, and getting the sandwich was inconvenient, to say the least. Yet, finally, no other tuna sandwich would do. I was obsessed. One day I took a long lunch and made the trek by bus. I got my sandwich, took it back to my desk, and started eating it really slowly, savoring every morsel. By the time I was halfway through, two things happened. One, I realized that the tuna itself wasn't very tasty at all. In fact, I could tell I was going to get indigestion if I finished the whole thing. Two, I remembered that it was during the time that I was falling in love with my husband that I had this sandwich for lunch practically every day. I knew what I'd really been 'missing' was not the sandwich but the feelings I'd had then. I'd felt carefree and on top of the world. Whereas lately I'd been anxious about whether having a child would put a damper on romance forever."

As for the notion that food cravings emanate from the baby itself, though there may be no way to prove it is true, this belief has been with us throughout history. Many cultures have had the notion that the mother's cravings are inextricably intertwined with the growing infant's desires or requirements, so much so that it is said babies are often born with birthmarks in the shape and color of the lusted-after food. (The French word *envie*, which means "birthmark," can also mean "craving.")[2]

At the very least, it is fun to think it might be true that our blossoming infant, who by six weeks is forming a jaw, mouth, and tiny dental buds, has definite preferences in matters of cuisine. Certainly, when it comes to food aversions, the flip side of the craving syndrome, women frequently hold to this theory. Many an expectant mother who discovers she is revolted by substances such as wine and coffee, which she'd imagined might prove difficult to give up, can be heard voicing the notion that her baby is making her "be good."

In sum, each theory of why a woman's tastes alter during

pregnancy can tell all or part of the story, and each new culinary preference may serve as a clue to one or more deeper needs. Whatever the reason, the fact is that drastic changes in food-related sensations prove an annoyance.

Expectant mothers often confess to being disgusted by even the most infinitesimal amounts of, say, garlic or parsley, onion or curry. People might try to talk them out of their emphatic "No thank you's" ("Oh, there's hardly any of *that* in this dish at all!"), but a pregnant woman cannot be dissuaded. She has no choice but to stand her ground, even if it means making a supper of unbuttered dinner rolls. And this "no choice" factor in and of itself is enough to cast her into a temporary funk.

Because the flip side of being suddenly, exquisitely, and brilliantly sensitive is that one is also suddenly vulnerable. Rather than feeling in charge of her dietary preferences, the expectant mother may feel at the mercy of her taste buds. And she may feel the same about her other sensory organs—for example, her nasal receptors.

What the Nose Knows

When we think of the senses, smell is often the last to be considered and the most likely to be undervalued. In fact, when evolution compelled humankind to rise and walk upright, many of smell's most seemingly practical uses seemed to go by the boards. Today we no longer employ our noses, distant from the ground as they are, for, say, tracking prey or sniffing out a suitable mate.

Or do we?

Recent research has been turning up some startling evidence that we are probably much more responsive to smell than we have supposed. In addition to our five million olfactory cells, humans, like many other mammals, have a tiny organ in the nasal cavity that responds to pheromones—natural substances that can trigger emotional responses such as anger, fear, and love.[3] It seems such sensitivity might influence our romantic inclinations after all. As for "tracking," contemporary marketers are convinced that our behavior as consumers is so influenced by scent that we might be prone to hunt down a particular automobile or dress to purchase because it exudes a particular aroma.[4]

One thing is for certain: You would not have to work very hard to convince a pregnant woman that the sense of smell is a probing and powerful one. The vast majority of mothers-to-be I spoke with reported experiencing new heights of aromatic pleasure, and repugnance, in the pregnant state. And a good many sounded as though they had developed a true case of hyperosmia (the official term for olfactory hypersensitivity), joking that they could probably sniff out a truffle from below the soil.

Why pregnancy breeds this sensual marvel none can say for certain. In fact, even *that* it exists cannot be said with utter certainty if one relies solely on controlled scientific experiments. While it's been borne out to researchers' satisfaction that females have a greater sensitivity to odors than males in general, no one has yet "proven" that pregnant females are keener sniffers than their nonpregnant sisters. But the anecdotal evidence is overwhelming. As one obstetrician said to me when I complained of smelling anything and everything, "Well, that means you're *good* and pregnant."

Some believe that a pregnant woman's high estrogen level is the likeliest instigator of acute smell-sensitivity. But perhaps it is part of Mother Nature's curriculum for Motherhood Preparedness 101. Experiments have shown that mothers can recognize the scent of their own children as early as the second day of birth.[5] Could pregnancy entail on-the-job training for this feat?

On a more esoteric note, it is true that, as both Freud and Darwin noted, the olfactory capacity of humans diminished with our species's "verticalization." The more "civilized" we became and the less crucial a sense of smell was to our survival, the less we relied upon it, and the less we tended to pay attention to it. But pregnancy is a time when a woman's body is in the business of carrying out the instructions of genetic coding that is billions of years old. It is as good a time as any to be thrust back in touch with the "earthier" aspects of our existence, and to feel somewhat humbled by their force.

Finally, on a more psychological note, smell is the sense most likely to revive memory. At times no more than a whiff of newly mowed lawn or fresh baked brownies can propel us into vivid reveries of childhood. During pregnancy, a natural part of the growth and change process is to reexperience certain aspects of our own upbringing. In this process our sense of smell can be one of our hardest-working allies.

Still, with smell, as with taste, the hypersensitivity pregnant women experience may be awfully distressing. As one woman recounted:

> "A couple of months after I got pregnant we moved into a new house that had wall-to-wall carpet already installed in the living room. That carpet had an odor that drove me wild. I couldn't exactly define it, but I could describe it. It was sort of a wet, sour smell, with undertones that were almost sulphurous. To me, it was very distinctive. Anyway, I must have tried six different rug cleaners and hired a professional cleaning service before I was satisfied that the odor was all gone. Meanwhile, my husband and I had more than a few cross words. He thought I was crazy. He said he never smelled a thing."

To the pregnant woman it suddenly may seem that compared to her everyone else has anosmia, an impaired ability to smell. And it's often those closest to her—friends, coworkers, most notably her spouse—who seem to have the biggest "blind spots" when it comes to perceiving the very odors that send her into a frenzy. To other people the pregnant woman's refined sensibilities may make her seem something of a prima donna. To her, those other people can seem boorishly oblivious.

Regardless of such discrepancies and divergencies, there is no reason to underestimate smell's effect on a pregnant woman's disposition, or to disrespect it. Anyone who is tempted to do so, should recall the words of two (presumably nonpregnant but nevertheless olfactorily sensitive) Frenchmen. As Montaigne said of odors, "I have often noticed that they make a change in me and work upon my spirits according to their properties."[6] And as Rousseau wrote, "The sense of smell is the sense of imagination; giving a stronger tone to the nerves, it greatly disturbs the brain."[7]

See No Evil, Hear No Evil

Taste and smell are both "contact senses" which induce chemical reactions in the body. The remaining three senses of sight, hearing, and touch can be thought of more as "mechanical senses." What we see, hear, and touch is, overall, somewhat less likely to be perceived subjectively. It's more common for two people to have differing opinions about whether or not something is too salty or smells sour, for example, than whether or not something is red or blue, hard or soft, or whether it sounds like a piano or a violin.

Nevertheless, perceiving nuance is critical to all the senses. And pregnant women seem to perceive greater degrees of subtlety even in the so-called mechanical realm. They are often more sensitive to, say, the flicker of a fluorescent light fixture, to the dull hum of an electrical appliance, or to a lump in the mattress. It is as if now that they are sharing their bodies with someone else they are doubly aware, twice as sentient as before, of what permeates the sensors of their eyes, ears, and skin.

A newfound finicky nature is only part of the pregnancy experience. What many pregnant women and their spouses recall is that the heightened sensitivity that dawned during the first trimester went beyond the senses and incorporated the sensibilities, i.e., the emotional permutations that the women underwent in response to the routine stimuli around them.

Take, for instance, the common daily practice of watching the evening news. It's astonishing just how many expectant mothers develop an aversion to this endeavor. As one said:

> "I simply couldn't bear to read or see stories about violence or war or, most especially, hunger. While I was pregnant, the U.S. was sending troops to Somalia to help with food distribution. This was a good thing, I thought. But I couldn't look at the footage. I was terrified I might have to confront the image of malnourished chil-

dren. Whenever the news came on I'd beg my husband to turn it off. If he was too caught up in it to oblige right away, I'd have to leave the room."

Take also the workaday occurrence of riding public transportation. Many mothers-to-be who prior to pregnancy did so as a matter of course often came to dread it. As one formerly intrepid New Yorker recalled:

"Riding the subway at rush hour became an ordeal early on. The screeching brakes, the unpleasant lighting, the oppressive underground air were bad enough. But the obscene graffiti really unnerved me. I obsessed on it. Why would someone do that? The look in people's eyes also got to me. Everyone looking deadpan, trying not to make contact. What kind of a world was this, I thought. Didn't anyone smile anymore?"

Foul language, heavy metal rock music, obnoxious morning deejays, car alarms, and pneumatic jackhammers may be among the least beloved sounds of the modern world to any reasonably discriminating adult. And everyone wishes, no doubt, that the glimpses of wrack and ruin which are wedged between commercials on the nightly news could be replaced by happier scenarios. But pregnant women seem to have a diminished ability to tolerate such fare. For better or worse, they simply don't wear blinders as effectively as most.

In a different place or time perhaps they wouldn't have had to be subjected to so much Sturm und Drang. In tribal societies, as Judith Goldsmith writes in her book *Childbirth Wisdom:* "Almost universally, the pregnant woman is protected from shocks, frights, and ugly sights."[8] And up through the eighteenth century, as Jacques Gélis writes in his *History of Childbirth,* textbooks warned that expectant mothers ought to be protected from such ills as "immoderate shouting" as well as "artillery and loud bells."[9] That no such preclusions are enforced in America today is, in a way, good news when one considers the politically incorrect ends such caveats might serve. But it is bad news when one considers how pregnant women—particularly before they begin to "show"—are often expected *by themselves as much or more than by everyone else* to carry on exactly as before, without acknowledgment that there is indeed much ado.

As a mother-to-be, you must realize that feeling more susceptible than usual to the sights and sounds, to the smell, touch, and taste of the world, is nothing to feel embarrassed about. In fact, nothing less is to be expected.

From the earliest weeks of pregnancy, your body is hard at work even if you or others don't yet recognize its invisible progress. By the eighth week of gestation it has manufactured all your baby's main internal organs. There is less energy available to serve as a buffer between you and the external world, not to mention less to shield you against your tumultuous inner emotions. Yet at the same time, because you have precious cargo on board you are intinctively attempting to insulate that cargo from displeasure and danger in all its forms. This is quite the noble mission, and quite the conflictful one. For it means you are charged with being a protector when you yourself may feel less safeguarded than ever before.

Still, there's a silver lining. For your very vulnerability can be a gateway to a type of knowledge with which we are not usually so in touch.

The Sixth Sense

Vulnerability is one of those loaded words, the use of which could be a bit misleading. In our society, where "the going gets tough and the tough get going," the term often connotes an unwelcome frailty. Yet there are certain aspects of being vulnerable which are enabling and enlightening, for to be vulnerable is also to be open and receptive.

Throughout the ages in various cultures it has often been supposed that being pregnant engenders enhanced intuitive and psychic capabilities. So far as I know, no one has yet designed an experiment to verify whether expectant mothers are genuinely more capable of empathic reactions to others or of so-called extrasensory perceptions than the average person. But here is another instance where anecdotal evidence and personal experience are compelling.

A number of pregnant women commented to me that their heightened sensitivities responded not just to the physical world. They felt better able to "pick up" on such things as the moods and intentions of people around them. As one said:

> "I could tell just by looking at someone whether they were sad or nervous, or even whether they were telling the truth or not. It wasn't as though I saw 'auras' or anything mystical like that. I don't even know if such things exist. But I can tell you I definitely 'sensed' their true attitudes."

It's often said that pregnant women are more absentminded, or "spacier" than usual. It's true! But this might lead one to conclude that they are using less of their brain power than they were before. Instead, we ought to acknowledge that to be pregnant is to avail oneself of a different way of knowing, a less linear and more integrated way. It's as if some fraction of the ninety percent of our brain power which allegedly goes untapped comes "on-line" with conception and expands with each passing month.

Speaking for myself, as a psychotherapist it is an integral part of my job to attempt to understand how my patients truly feel about something, and to discern the real meaning behind their words, even if they are not yet consciously aware of it. Through years of training and practice, I have worked at honing these skills and applying them with some success. But while I was pregnant, such work was far more effortless. With greater speed, I could pick up on subtleties of emotional demeanor. With greater frequency than what had been typical for me, I could silently predict what might be said *before* it was said aloud. And if what was verbalized was not entirely truthful, it was as if a bell would sound in my head.

Who knows what makes the pregnant woman more perceptive than ever. Is it that, along with her increased ability to smell actual odors, she can, as the idioms have it, "smell a rat" if someone is being dishonest, or tell if something "fishy" is going on? Anatomist David Berliner, a biotechnology researcher formerly of the University of Utah, has shown that the tiny organ in our nasal cavity which actively responds to pheromones can detect nearly a dozen different chemicals produced by the human skin.[10] If, as is suspected, we humans exhibit a different chemical balance according to mood (when depressed, for example, or when we're anxiously trying to conceal a truth), perhaps this is what pregnant women are "sniffing out." Just a speculation, though this could account for the expectant mother's perspicaciousness. Or maybe the expectant mother is simply open enough—"vulnerable" enough, if you will—to tune into things that all humankind might tune into if only we disciplined ourselves to make the attempt on a regular basis.

Mourning Sickness

So being vulnerable is not all bad. If one is curious enough and introspective enough, it could be quite a boon. Still, no rumination on first trimester sensations would be complete without a mention of a special yet commonplace condition which can make women feel vulnerable in not-so-wonderful ways. Morning sickness—the inaccurately named nausea that can actually affect a pregnant woman at any time of day—is a circumstance that makes some women feel helpless and beleaguered.

Not everyone is given to so-called morning sickness in the early months of pregnancy. And of those who are, some experience only minor, or mercifully brief, bouts of queasiness. But others have different tales to tell, and a common theme runs through them:

> "I felt alarmed that my body was so *out of control*. I used to do everything I could think of to keep from throwing up, because that is another out of control feeling."

> "I felt that since I wasn't showing, everything should be 'normal.' Every day I told myself I should be feeling better by now, and wondered what was wrong with me. *I felt I had no say in my life* and that I was being taken over by mysterious forces."

"Instead of focusing on the life that was growing inside me, I felt like an invalid. I had a sense of *stepping to the side of my own life,* of not being able to participate."

The common theme here is a sense of disempowerment. When a woman has intense and lengthy bouts of morning sickness, she can experience herself as defenseless—impotent, if you will. Moreover she may see herself as "botching" the job of expectant motherhood. Feeling ill, she might believe she is ill-suited for the task at hand. Along with this there is often a sense of being unfairly treated by the universe. Why, she wants to know, are these debilitating episodes befalling her when all she is trying to do is have a happy, healthy baby?

Alas, as with so many women's health issues, not as much research has been done into the matter as one would hope. Many possible factors are suspected of contributing to morning sickness. Among them are low blood sugar, B-complex deficiencies, changes in the production of digestive enzymes and stomach acids, and, of course, the adjustment to increased hormone production.[11] But no one seems quite certain how all this adds up to create a specific gastrointestinal syndrome.

Similarly, no entirely satisfactory explanation has ever been given which accounts for the unusual fact that in some non-Western societies (notably Eskimo and African tribes and Oriental cultures other than the Japanese), what we refer to as morning sickness is not a common complaint. Some attribute this strange discrepancy to differences in the diet of Westerners and non-Westerners. Others cite the Western high-stress lifestyle, and the fatigue it induces, as the culprit behind first trimester nausea. And some with a bent for cultural anthropology suspect that Western women contract morning sickness because it is part of our belief system that pregnancy and first trimester nausea go hand in hand. Where there is no expectation that this will happen, they say, it does not happen.

As with sensory phenomena, people do believe that psychological factors play a role. But here is an ironic twist. Unfortunately, some of those who advance the theory that morning sickness is psychologically engendered offer only the glibbest sort of cause and effect. An expectant mother throws up, they say, when deep down she really "wants to be rid of the baby."

Beware such smug pronouncements. Such reasoning is misleading and oversimplified. (As you already know, having mixed feelings is common and natural and does *not* mean you aren't committed to the pregnancy and the baby.) Such pronouncements are also destructive. Needless to say, many already nauseated pregnant women who hear it will feel further nauseated, for they are, in effect, being told to swallow massive amounts of guilt along with their soda crackers.

Happily, there is another psychologically oriented theory that is more palatable. I call it the "mourning sickness" theory. It purports that if indeed some part of a woman's nausea is unconsciously inspired, it is likely because there is something in her life—perhaps some aspect of a relationship, some pattern of behavior, or some now outmoded way of thinking—that will no longer serve her as she readies herself to give birth and to mother. Subliminally she may know this, but consciously she may not. That is why Ann Fuller, a midwife who also trains labor coaches and childbirth educators in the San Francisco Bay area, asks her patients afflicted with morning sickness, "What is not working in your life that you need to 'throw up'?"

If you are one of the many, many women who are beleaguered by morning sickness, this could be a good question to ask yourself. Your answers may surprise you. You could find, for example, that you wish to be free of particular residues of your own childhood, or of annoying or disappointing aspects of your relationship with your spouse or with your parents. Perhaps, as you prepare for the awesome duties of motherhood, there is an aspect of your own personality that is disturbing you and that you would like to "throw up" and cast off. If so, gaining an awareness of this may help you put your subliminal impulses into words, instead of somatic actions. In talking with someone you trust, you can unburden yourself. And in unburdening yourself you can "mourn"—without literally throwing up—whatever it is you need to relinquish in order to get on with the business of pregnancy.

A caution, however. Don't expect overnight miracles from this process, since it could well take a while, if indeed it works for you. And, as Fuller suggests, women are in a better frame of mind for coming to terms with any psychological bugaboos that may be contributing to morning sickness *after* they've begun to alleviate their physical symptoms.

So do try the remedies that your prenatal caregiver recommends and that seem to make sense to you. Indeed many of them can help you manage your pregnancy well even after the first trimester (such as eating small meals throughout the day, carrying high protein snacks, and not waiting until you are very hungry before you start to eat). But do not neglect to ask yourself if anything is bothering you that you have yet to acknowledge (even if morning sickness is ultimately not its indicator).

And while you are at it, whether you have morning sickness or not, do not neglect the following:

❖ AN EXPECTANT MOTHER'S PRIVILEGES AND PREROGATIVES

Slow down. Though for many busy women this will fall into the "easier said than done" category, it cannot be said emphatically enough how imperative this is. By the second month of pregnancy your body is busy "moonlighting," nurturing the new life inside you. Correspondingly, you are being sensually bombarded. Give yourself a break—even a little one if that's all you can manage or all you can tolerate—to rest during the day. If you can't nap or meditate, then simply sitting quietly and paging through a magazine is fine. If you don't do this, you will be accumulating a physical and emotional deficit.

Solicit and accept a helping hand on the home front. You may have mixed feelings about certain people's solicitousness toward you. On the job, for example, it may be unnerving to you to be treated differently, even if differently means deferentially. So if you want to go on with business as usual at this stage, and can, fine. But home is another story. As much as it's possible for you temperamentally and logistically, allow yourself to be pampered. If your husband offers to cook and clean more than he usually does, let him. (So much the better for avoiding many of the odors you find objectionable.) And if he doesn't offer, help him think of the suggestion. Likewise, if you already have children old enough to make themselves useful, encourage them to do so.

Heed and honor the warnings of your senses. Trust your instincts and never fight what your senses seem to be telling you. If you find something distasteful to eat, don't eat it. If a food or an aroma or a sound offends or irritates you, see if it's possible to get it away from you. If not, try getting away from it.

Insulate yourself and your child in a "mind exercise." If none of the above is possible or practical, employ visualization techniques to armor yourself against unpleasantness. Picture a bubble of light surrounding you, one that negativity simply bounces off of. When in circumstances where you feel threatened, uneasy, or uncomfortable remind yourself that your bubble is impenetrable. You and your baby are safe.

Seek out the positive. In the Middle Ages pregnant women visited shrines of the Virgin Mary. In early modern Europe they made their way to various sanctuaries at special moments in the liturgical year.[12] Many of us have no opportunity for such pilgrimages, or no inclination. But we can undertake some shorter journeys to calm and comfort ourselves. Now that you are more sensually alert than ever, take advantage of that fact and seek out places and experiences that make you feel tranquil and composed. Whether you choose to find respite in churches and synagogues, or gardens, museums, or symphony halls, is a matter of individual preference. The point is to surround yourself with what is soothing and pleasurable as much as possible.

Even if this is not your first pregnancy, do what is necessary to find the time to enjoy it!

Add your memories to your journal. Your heightened sensitivity will serve to evoke many memories for you at this time, probably some good and some not so good, and these will be added to your emotional stew. One way to process the memories and allow them to serve you rather than unnerve you is to keep track of them in your pregnancy journal. If you find yourself having "flashbacks" of childhood or of past pregnancies or past relationships, write about them and how they make you feel. Ask yourself why they have come up at this time and what they can teach you.

Network. Now that you have had some time to process the fact that you are well and truly pregnant, it is time to begin engaging in this most important of tasks. No matter where you live or what you do, make it your business to talk to other pregnant women and compare notes. You will be thrilled to know that what you are experiencing is being experienced by others as well.

This is not a time for isolation but for connection. Most pregnant women are itching to talk about what they're experiencing and it's likely any small overture on your part will be eagerly received and reciprocated.

Your finely tuned senses, all six of them, are extremely important tools. If you respect the information they provide, they can steer you in the right direction in more ways than one. Perhaps one of the most important ways they can guide you is in helping you select the kind of prenatal and birth care that is right for you. This is the subject of the next chapter. And even if you already think you know whom you want to administer care and attend the birth of your child, please don't skip it. For there is much to consider, perhaps more than you thought.

3 Steering Through the System

We are too often treated like babies having babies
when we should be in training, like acolytes, novices
to high priestesses, like serious applicants for the
space program.

—LOUISE ERDRICH
"A Woman's Work"

*By the start of the third month of pregnancy the baby inside
me weighed less than a kumquat. Nevertheless his face was
taking on recognizably human characteristics and he was already beginning to exercise his tiny muscles. I was awestruck
by these facts, as I was by the reality that what was happening
to my body was as old as humankind itself. Yet to my obstetrician, it was more or less business as usual.*

*My monthly prenatal checkups paid no homage to miracles
and allowed little time to ponder the mystery of it all. Instead,
every four weeks or so, along with suffering the usual indignities
of stirrups, paper gowns, and plastic urine sample cups, I was
subjected to high-tech procedures meant to assure me, and
everyone concerned, that things were proceeding smoothly. In
a way I was grateful that the vigilance was so keen, and that
problems had the potential of being spotted and treated before
they threatened the pregnancy. But I also felt strangely dissatisfied. I had the odd sense that I was simultaneously being protected and invaded, attended to and neglected.*

To complicate matters, my obstetrician, who had been recommended by a friend who'd known him as a solo practitioner, informed me he was now part of a group practice. Office policy mandated that he rotate shifts with two colleagues, each of whom I'd have to see in turn, and any one of which might deliver my baby. The first doctor I met seemed reasonably pleasant and accessible enough. The second, though clearly efficient and knowledgeable, struck me as emotionally cold. It didn't help that the nursing staff already had me lying supine on an exam table when I was introduced to her. This was one indignity too many.

After lengthy internal debate, much research, and several conversations with my husband, I opted to make a change. Since we'd already decided to move out of the city in anticipation of family life, I decided to switch my prenatal care to our new locale near the New Jersey shore. There I found a very experienced, reassuring, and easygoing certified nurse midwife who worked in an obstetrical practice. She allowed the time to answer my questions, and when I said things like, "Hey, I'm nervous," or "I'm pretty blue this week," she did not simply respond, "That's common," or "That's hormones," and show me the door. She soothed me, joked with me, understood me. Indeed my visits with her were so informative, so calming, and so much fun I wished they could go on and on. I wanted to talk about the intricacies of my pregnancy forever. But, of course, there was always someone else in the waiting room. And I was still wearing a paper gown. Such is the nature of the maternity care system, but at least I had found a niche in it that worked pretty well for me. . . .

Biology and Technology

By the third month of pregnancy, if not even sooner, women are generally looking to settle the question of who will administer the balance of their prenatal care and oversee the birth of their child. For some, the question is easily settled. Perhaps they have a good relationship with an obstetrician who has also given them gynecological care, or with a midwife with whom they have been through a previous pregnancy. Perhaps, through the grapevine, they find someone with whom they "click" right off. That practitioner will be diligent in looking after the health and well-being of the developing baby but equally as diligent in communicating with and listening to the mother-to-be, and in treating her as what she is: *a unique individual undergoing and responding to an ancient process in her own particular way.*

For others, though, finding a practitioner with whom they can establish a good rapport is a challenge. And too often they feel they must settle for something less than they'd hoped for. No small number of mothers-to-be I spoke with confided their dissatisfaction with the emotional tenor of their prenatal care. Ironically many believe the more sophisticated the technical level of the prenatal care the more "bedside manner" seems to be forfeited.

Some say this is a sign of our society's unconsciously trying to separate sexuality and plain old down and dirty humanity from the birth process. Others suggest that the medical establishment has a vested interest, in terms of economics and power, in surrounding a natural process with professional mumbo jumbo. But Perri Klass, a well-known Harvard-trained physician and author, provided an insider's perspective when she recounted her passage through a year of medical school while she herself was pregnant.

As Klass writes: "In our reproductive medicine course, the emphasis was on the abnormal, the pathological. . . . We learned nothing about any of the problems encountered in a normal pregnancy . . . We learned nothing about the emotional aspects of pregnancy, nothing about helping women prepare for labor and delivery. In other words, none of my medical school classmates would have been capable of answering even the most basic questions about pregnancy asked by people in my [lay] childbirth class.[1]

When Klass mentioned this to her own doctor, he agreed that normal childbirth was not sufficiently honored in the curriculum. It seems that in the busy, high-tech world of today's medicine, there is simply little time for, and little interest in, the blessedly ordinary. And while the emphasis in training obstetrical medical personnel to manage complications during pregnancy has some obvious and important advantages, to focus *solely* on such matters has far-reaching psychological disadvantages.

The good news is that in recent years, more and more expectant mothers have begun to define themselves as consumers of medical services rather than passive patients. They want to work with practitioners who can give them what they want and treat them as they wish to be treated. And though it often takes a bit of effort, they are finding them.

The bad news is that once a woman starts to look around for options she may feel confused and pressured, especially if this is her first pregnancy. With all the conflicting advice and philosophies around, and with little or no experience in being a proactive medical consumer (for most of us have grown up following "doctor's orders" and questioning nothing), it can be difficult to discover exactly what it is she wants.

Hence, the first rule of thumb for those who would counsel, "Physician, heal thyself," is "Consumer, now thyself."

Knowing Thyself

Virtually every woman wants to work with an obstetrician or midwife who is respectful, concerned, and compassionate. But beyond that, just who is the ideal practitioner? Is it one who provides the expectant mother with the feeling that he will take care of everything and that there is no need to worry, or one who gives her the feeling that *she* is in control and that he is only there to assist and support as necessary? Is it one who goes over in painstaking detail what hazards to avoid for the sake of her growing baby, or one who takes a more casual approach? Is it one who assures her her fears are common, or one who cracks a good joke to try to diffuse those fears?

The answer is, it depends.

What a woman needs from a doctor or midwife on an emotional level is a very personal matter. Regardless of what her friends or relatives tell her, or regardless of what is trendy, she must make up her own mind as to what approach makes her feel secure, valued, and understood. The bottom line is that no matter how many accusatory fingers one points at the medical system, it's impossible to achieve *any* satisfaction in it at all without being introspective and honest with oneself.

Here, for example, is how two different women recounted their experience with the very same obstetrician (let's call him Dr. X), a thorough and impeccably credentialed physician with an avuncular, joshing manner, who let his patients know early on that, in his opinion, modern science had made pregnancy and childbirth far easier to cope with than at any time in history, and that the best way to remain low risk was to do just as he advised. Though he endorsed childbirth that was "awake and aware," he maintained that labor would probably proceed most smoothly if they agreed to the episiotomies and epidurals he routinely recommended to "speed things along" and minimize pain. To patients who said they wanted totally natural childbirth he winked and said, "Whatever you like, but I bet when the time comes you'll say, 'Ouch, Doc, hurry up with those drugs!' "

> "This guy made me a little mad," said 29-year-old Francine. "Yes, he was personable, but I found him patronizing. I felt his real attitude was that he would 'rescue' me from the 'dangers' of pregnancy and childbirth and that I ought to feel dependent on him. I don't enjoy feeling dependent on authority figures. He also made me a little uneasy. I thought his proposed interventions during childbirth would deprive me of the full experience, and although he said I could do as I liked, so long as there was no danger to myself or the baby, I had the sinking feeling that he would nudge me in the direction of medication if I started to feel anxious and afraid. And, knowing how I am when I feel vulnerable, I might just give in unless I had someone there to encourage me in the other direction."

> "[Dr. X] made me feel safe," said 32-year-old Robin. "I have always felt so scared of actually giving birth to a baby that I almost decided not to have children at all. But now I felt like I was in good hands, and that he wasn't going to let any harm come to me. I

liked feeling that he was scrutinizing everything and being really cautious. To me he seemed like a 'good father' type. I also like that he made me laugh, which relaxed me."

Is one of these women being foolish or unreasonable? No, the two of them are just being themselves. They are different and need different things in order to feel comfortable.

Francine is averse to dependency, which she felt Dr. X fostered. Also, for her, the satisfaction of childbirth was tied into not missing out on anything. Hence, she did not value what Dr. X said he had to offer. Knowing enough about herself to realize that her commitment to a birth with little or no technological intervention might waver under pressure, she ultimately opted for care by a practitioner who made her feel more in control and who voiced the conviction that, barring complications, the safest, simplest childbirth was a medication-free childbirth.

Robin, on the other hand, was calmed by Dr. X. For her, the perceived risk and pain of childbearing was strong. Having a "good father" figure to help her through seemed psychologically essential. She was comforted by knowing that her pregnancy and childbirth would follow the ritualized path prescribed by modern medicine. She found solace in the thought that she would not have to suffer the way she imagined women suffered in the 'old days' and thanked her lucky stars she had found someone who could, if not put her fears entirely to rest, at least abate them.

It's not at all uncommon to find that a practitioner who soothes one woman scares another. And the same is true when it comes to methods of childbirth.

Consider, for example, the disparate reactions of three women who attended an orientation at a freestanding birthing center which boasted a homelike environment and which wholeheartedly embraced a philosophy of natural childbirth and family participation. Here, good prenatal care was considered to be a joint venture between the expectant mother and her caregivers. The births at this center were attended by highly qualified midwives, with backup transfers to hospitals arranged when necessary.

"I felt this was a caring place," said 31-year-old Avery. "They treated pregnant women like adults. The staff made me feel my needs and desires were important. After speaking with the capable and encouraging midwives, any skepticism I had disappeared. I had found a place where I felt I could take charge of my child's debut in the world. As a mother-to-be that was of paramount importance to me. Besides, I've always tended to do things in a slightly unconventional way. That's just who I am and how I think."

"I felt this was a frightening environment," said 26-year-old Eileen. "I didn't *want* to be somewhere that looked like a home, I wanted to be somewhere that looked, you know, professional. My grandmother delivered at home. Wasn't this a step backwards? Besides, when I listened to the staff they sounded unrealistic. I felt so much could go wrong. And I knew there would be pain no matter what. The more they talked about how beautiful and sacred childbirth was, the more I kept wondering if they knew what they were doing. I hightailed it back to a conventional obstetrical practice."

"I really liked the feeling I got from the midwives at the birthing center," said 25-year-old Beth. "They made me believe I would be strong and capable throughout pregnancy and childbirth. I found their attitude uplifting. It was like we were all on a par, endeavoring to do something wonderful and challenging together. My problem was that my husband, who accompanied me, was truly nervous about worst-case scenarios. He wanted to be supportive, and would have gone along with me, but I knew he would not totally be able to get over his fears of my having to be moved to a hospital during labor if something got complicated. No statistic about the safety of birthing centers and backup transports would convince him deep down.

I considered him a full partner in this endeavor. Besides, I felt I couldn't bear him being so stressed out because I knew that would stress *me* out. It wasn't worth it. So we ended up finally arranging prenatal care with a nurse midwife who would help me give birth at an ABC (Alternative Birthing Center) located on hospital premises. Under the circumstances, this seemed like the best of all worlds."

Once again, we see how feelings of support and security can be quite subjective. What empowered the independent-minded Avery traumatized the more conservative Eileen. And though the conventionally inclined could argue endlessly with more nonconformist types about the wisdom of the choices these expectant mothers ultimately made, the point is that they understood themselves well enough to do what most suited their personalities. As for Beth, who opted for a compromise approach out of concern for her husband's feelings, it is to her credit that she understood the dynamics of her marriage well enough to predict that ongoing anxiety in her husband would induce intolerable anxiety in her. Given that, the middle road she embarked on made good sense and freed her and her spouse to get on with the business of looking confidently forward together.

Along with their self-knowledge, all of these mothers-to-be shared the traits of open-mindedness and curiosity. None of them were passive and all were willing to explore options. Such exploration is critical. For no matter what anyone tells you about who should or shouldn't administer your prenatal care and about what type of birth you should or shouldn't consider, your choice cannot be a "wrong" choice *as long as it is an informed choice.*

Getting the Facts

The International Childbirth Education Association publishes two invaluable documents. The first, *The Pregnant Patient's Bills of Rights*, helps expectant mothers understand the standards of care to which they are entitled. The second equally important document is called *The Pregnant Patient's Responsibilities*. It lists an expectant mother's obligations to herself and her unborn child so that she can maximize her chances of having a healthy and satisfying experience of pregnancy and childbirth. Its first precept is: "The Pregnant Patient is responsible for learning about the physical and psychological process of labor, birth, and postpartum recovery. The better informed expectant parents are, the better they will be able to participate in decisions concerning the planning of their care."[2]

One can hardy go wrong to live by these words from the moment one's pregnancy is a known fact—and even earlier if one is knowingly planning a family. But whatever point you have reached in your own pregnancy by now, it is never too late to begin educating yourself.

In theory, one can never be too informed, but realistically everyone has time limitations. So perhaps the most efficient way to tackle pregnancy and childbirth education is to divide it into two stages: armchair work and legwork.

First, even if you think you know exactly what you want (perhaps because all your friends saw such and such a practitioner or had a such and such type of delivery), you should learn what is available. This is the armchair phase. Even a couple of hours spent perusing books and articles at a library can begin to tell you a great deal about such issues as the potential risks and benefits of various medical procedures during pregnancy and childbirth and what alternatives may be available.

Once you believe you have an idea of what type of approach is right for you, you can delve more deeply (while still remaining in your armchair) by reading further and by talking to people who have experienced that approach.

Next, you'll need to discern exactly who is most likely to give you the kind of care you want and collaborate with you in preparing for the sort of birth you would prefer. Another few hours making phone inquiries to local hospitals, doctors' offices, midwives, birthing centers, and childbirth educators can narrow the field. At this point, the second phase, involving legwork and face-to-face interviewing, can begin.

Though being the one to *ask* the questions during a medical visit may feel a little weird, it is not only appropriate, but extremely wise to ask potential caregivers, in a nonconfrontational but firm way, such questions as:

❖ How long do you allow for a routine prenatal visit?
❖ Who is likely to actually be in attendance at my child's birth?

- Who are your backups and how can I get to know them?
- Can I deliver with minimal intervention, if there are no complications and if that's what I should choose?
- Will my husband be welcome at prenatal visits and in the delivery room?

For anyone who is especially concerned with some specific issues, it's also perfectly reasonable to pose such questions as:

- What pain medications do you generally recommend, should I desire or require any?
- What is your rate of c-section deliveries, and under what circumstances would you perform them?
- What percentage of your birth mothers receive episiotomies, and under what circumstances would you perform them?

A woman who knows herself and who listens carefully to the responses to such questions should have little trouble determining whether a particular practitioner is right for her. If she is the sort of woman who values very highly getting to know—and being known by—the person who will guide her through pregnancy and birth, she will know, for example, that a doctor who schedules prenatal visits ten minutes apart and who shows little sensitivity about which of his or her associates may be delivering the baby is not for her. If she places a high value on having a vaginal birth, she will not wind up with an obstetrician who has a twenty-five percent cesarian rate. And if she places a high value on being talked to in a noncondescending manner, she will certainly not end up with a practitioner who sniffs at her questions and rushes her out the door.

But even once an expectant mother is certain she has what she wants and feels content with her choice, a hurdle remains. She must resist the forces of those who would try to dissuade her.

The Rhetoric Factor

Most expectant mothers say they desire the same things when it comes to the birth of their children. They want to be as physically comfortable as it is possible to be during labor and delivery. And they want the safest possible outcome for themselves and their babies. But there are differing schools of thought as to how to accomplish these ends.

One school believes that the best bet for minimizing pain and keeping mother and child safe is to let the doctor and hospital staff do what is conventional and use high-tech medical procedures from fetal monitors to IV's to pain relievers. The other believes that the surest road to these goals is completely "natural" childbirth. (One could argue that all childbirth is natural, but this term has come to connote a birth which bypasses all medical interventions.)

Where one school says, "Lie back," the other says, "Squat." Where one says, "Have the episiotomy and get it over with," the other says, "Perineum massage will do the trick." And where one says, "Have the epidural, for God's sake," the other says, "Just learn to breathe and relax to manage contractions."

At some point in her research, the self-educated consumer will come across arguments for both sides. Both may seem convincing and compelling, and she may decide to adopt a wait-and-see attitude, postponing certain decisions, such as whether or not to have an epidural block, until she is in the throes of labor and sees how her body and psyche are reacting. But by making a decision as to *who* will help her give birth to her child and *where* that birth will take place, she is inevitably beginning to ally herself with one school or the other.

In the polarized world of childbirth as it now exists in America, she will likely find that she has not only allied herself with a group of people who share ideas about what constitutes a reasonable way to approach the physical challenges of labor, but also with a group of people who share particular political tenets. (Not "political" in the sense of being Democrats or Republicans, but in the sense of embracing or challenging the status quo.) Though joining any such cadre may have been the farthest thing from her mind, she may now be considered "one of them" by the "other side."

If she heads toward a goal of natural childbirth, she may find herself needled by people who espouse the virtues of the medical establishment, and who may regard her, at best, as letting herself in for a lot of unnecessary discomfort and, at worst, potentially threatening the well-being of her newborn.

If, on the other hand, she chooses a routine hospital delivery with all of its standard rituals and accoutrements, she may find herself branded by natural childbirth advocates as someone who will foolishly deprive herself of a peak life experience. At best, they may say, this expectant mother is letting herself in for a lot of unnecessary discomfort, and, at worst, she is—you guessed it—potentially threatening the well-being of her newborn.

Technology over nature! Nature over technology! So the rhetoric goes . . . and goes. Women who select birthing situations at the far end of the spectrum are most at risk for being outrightly rebuked, whether they are among those who choose a technological birth with all the trimmings or among the three percent who choose freestanding birthing centers or the one percent who choose home births.[3]

> "When I told some of my more unconventional friends that I had faith in my doctor, who had delivered my two older sisters in standard high-tech form and left them very satisfied, and that I, for one, couldn't wait to have my epidural," recalls 26-year-old Cara, "they professed horror. They said, 'You have been brainwashed!' "

> "When I told my relatives and coworkers that I was planning on a home birth you would have thought I'd said I was going to fly to the moon to have my baby," said 32-year-old Deanne. "They couldn't begin to comprehend my well thought out reasons for this, and they did not believe my midwife and I knew what we were doing. They kept telling me I should have been grateful to have been born in a time when women no longer *had* to have babies at home. 'You're a throwback,' they said."

But a few are exempt from critiques. Even those who steer toward a middle course (such as the hospital-based Alternative Birthing Center) may find that what they view as a reasonable compromise incites warnings and judgment calls from both sides of the debate.

"Here I thought I was opting for the best of two worlds," said 34-year-old Yvette, "in choosing an ABC which was literally right down the hall from all the high-tech equipment anyone could want in an emergency. But now everyone had a warning for me. Some people said, 'You're making this ten times as hard on yourself. *Just go down the hall and get the drugs.*' Others said, 'Stay out of the hospital all together. *Once they've got you, they'll take over your baby's birth.*' "

Such rhetoric, unsolicited and annoying though it may be, can nonetheless be intimidating and could lead to second-guessing oneself. Expectant mothers must be stalwart in their intention to do what, after due consideration, they believe is correct for them. They ought to be especially wary of anyone employing the following rhetorical devices:

SCARE STORIES: Employed most often by the technically inclined to persuade the naturally inclined, these frightening anecdotes are meant to accentuate the perceived dangers of a nonmainstream birthing option. They usually begin with the phrase, "This happened to my sister-in-law's cousin . . ." and end with, "If she hadn't been hooked up to the [insert latest medical gadget of your choice] I shudder to think what would have happened!"

CULTURAL CONFUSIONS: Employed most often by the naturally inclined to persuade the technically inclined, these anecdotes dwell on the remarkable ease and preternatural calm with which women in tribal societies give birth under trees, only to return, moments later, to whip up a batch of yam porridge for the family's dinner.

Both types of stories are usually exaggerated, if not intentionally then as a result of the "playing telephone" effect, where tales grow taller and taller as they are passed further and further from their original source. What truth there is in the tales is relative, anyhow. For example, while it may be true that being hooked up to such and such a gadget may have been extremely beneficial to so-and-so's sister-in-law's cousin, her circumstances may have been vastly different from those of the woman at whom this bit of rhetoric is being aimed.

Likewise, it is indeed true that birth in tribal societies is often a significantly different sort of experience than it is in the late twentieth-century United States. But while we could all learn some beneficial things from the tribal woman's approach to pregnancy and childbirth (some of which will be cited in this book), it must also be remembered that, as Sheila Kitzinger writes, "In every culture birth is a socially constructed event."[4] The tribal woman meets her birth experience with a different set of expectations and a far narrower range of choices than does the average American. She is also under tremendous social and psychological pressure to make a great show of her bravery in childbirth. As Dr. Melvin Konner, a field anthropologist turned physican, wrote of his experience among the !Kung San (the bushmen hunter-gatherers of Africa's Kalahari): "Women conceptualized birth as an almost ritual trial of physical courage."[5] Such is the way in the tribal woman's world. If any expectant mother in our society wants to follow in her path, that is her right. And she may well get a great deal out of it. But it is also her right to opt for a hospital bed and a Demerol drip.

All in all, an expectant woman needs to stand firm in the face of the friends and acquaintances who would attempt to alter her chosen childbirth course. But, of course, when it comes to coercion, nearly everyone wants to get into the act. So, lastly but not least, a word should be said here about dealing with someone who may vocalize her opinions very strongly—the expectant mother's mother again.

Does Mother Know Best?

Unfortunately, many of us who are of childbearing age had mothers who experienced childbirth from the vantage point of "twilight sleep." A powerful anesthetic (part morphine, part scopolamine) rendered them unconscious from early in labor until after delivery. Dr. Joseph B. DeLee, who described the procedure in 1940, said: "The object is to maintain the patient in a state of amnesia . . . Care must be given that the woman does not attain full consciousness."[6] Women who gave birth in this fashion (and a "fashion" it was, passed down from the wealthy who traveled to Germany for this sort of birth in the 1930s and then eagerly embraced by American obstetrics in the midst of a busy post-war baby boom), have no clear memory of childbirth, except as something they thought should be dreaded and avoided to the extent it was possible to do.

What recollections they do have are often of humiliating experiences that had to do with hospital personnel ordering them about, treating them like infants themselves, and declining to provide them with any information as to what was going on. (My own mother recalls a nurse climbing atop her and pressing a knee into her stomach in order to push out the placenta without so much as an "Excuse me," never mind an explanation.)

Not surprisingly, many of these women have negative associations with childbirth. To them, what little they recalled was bad enough. To endure any more without benefit of a chemical fog must be, they assume, even worse. Hence, no matter what choice a daughter makes in this day and age when "awake and aware" is the general rule even for most of those who opt for high-tech births, she may be faced with a mother who shakes her head, clucks her tongue, and conveys the message that this is sheer madness. (More than one woman I spoke with recalled their mothers saying words to the effect, "Why anyone would want to be awake for *that* I'll never understand.")

A daughter who voices any desire to undergo childbirth in an unconventional manner may come up against a truly hysterical mother exclaiming that no grandchild of *hers* is going to be born in such a dangerous venue. In fact, she forbids it!

> "When I told my mother I was doing a lot of looking around and was considering having natural birth at a freestanding birthing clinic, she flipped," said 28-year-old Sharon. "She literally said to me, 'If you do anything like that to *my grandchild* I'll . . . I'll have a heart attack. And then who will you get to baby-sit?' "

Though it is extremely difficult to cope with such strong opinions on the part of one's mother, and though pregnant women may well wish to avoid such emotionally charged outbursts, this sort of maternal coercion ought not hold sway. Chances are, mothers who are most upset by their daughters' choices of prenatal care and childbirth plans are those who had the least information and the fewest options when they themselves were bearing children. Offering a mother as much objective information as possible concerning one's choice—explaining why it is both safe and sane—is all a pregnant daughter can do. It should help. But, in any case, a mother-to-be must do what makes her and her spouse comfortable, and make a concerted effort not to let her mother's fears, understandable though they may be, become her own.

Testing, Testing

Even after selecting a practitioner and beginning to plan toward a particular birth locale, a pregnant woman still has some important medical decisions to make by her third month of pregnancy. These revolve around what sort of prenatal tests she will have administered, for example, ultrasound, chorionic villi sampling, alpha-fetoprotein screening, and amniocentesis.

When it comes to the physical aspects of these tests, the pros and cons may be fairly cut-and-dry. Statistics can tell a woman what her chances are, given her age, family history and so forth, of bearing a child with a particular birth defect. And though there is some debate, they can also tell her to some extent what the odds are that the test itself will do her baby any harm. But what statistics cannot tell her is the emotional impact—positive, negative, or mixed—the tests will have on her and on her feelings about her growing baby.

Many women consider these tests a pathway to bonding with their unborn children. Ultrasound in particular, which can be done on its own or as a prelude to amniocentesis, has been hailed by many mothers-to-be (and fathers-to-be) as a magnificent opportunity to "see" their babies and make what some describe as an instantaneous emotional connection with them. Some women even report an improved ability to stick to prenatal diet and health regimes once a sonogram helps them "get acquainted" with their growing children. There is now a perceptible incentive to avoid the sweets, abstain from the glass of wine, and so on.

Many also feel that test results which tell them all is well help them relax for the balance of their pregnancies. Knowing their babies are developing normally prevents them from dwelling on certain fears, they say, and even cuts down on the number of anxious dreams they are having.

These are obvious potential emotional benefits that may result from undergoing prenatal testing. However, there are potential emotional "downsides" as well.

For example, some women are reluctant to believe fully in the viability of their pregnancies until various tests are completed and the results are in. During this period of enforced delay a woman may defer feelings of attachment to a baby whose future she regards as uncertain. And carrying a life inside her she is unable to wholly commit to can be a source of dissonance and stress. (As one expectant mother recalled, "I willfully reined my happiness in until the doctor said, in effect, it was okay to be optimistic.")

Also, some feel the testing procedures themselves are so anxiety-provoking that they can hardly bear to contemplate them. It's rare indeed to meet a woman who doesn't wince when it is first explained to her how amniotic fluid is obtained. And a few react quite strongly to the image. ("I lost weeks of sleep thinking about a needle being poked into my tummy," confided one mother-to-be.) If they go through with the process, it is at least at a temporary cost to their equanimity. (I know one woman who clutched her arms above her head so tightly during an amniocentesis that her muscles hurt for weeks afterward.) And even afterward, if a woman finds out the good news that her baby is fine, she may lie awake wondering if the test itself initiated any harmful effects.

Other women feel the process of intuition is belittled by an overreliance on medical tests. There are women whose instincts tell them that theirs are happy, healthy babies. Should they put themselves through the stressful testing rituals, they wonder, to confirm what they already feel they know on a visceral level? And is this just a way, they complain, of reinforcing female helplessness? And finally, some feel that to have prenatal testing is tantamount to questioning their faith. It violates their sense of trust in Divine Providence, and that trust is precisely what sees them through adversity.

Needless to say, none of these opinions can be labeled right or wrong. Once again, knowing oneself, knowing one's options, and refusing to be coerced out of doing what feels right for oneself and one's baby will serve an expectant mother well.

A woman's being attuned to her own feelings and values will help signify what kinds of procedures would tend to make her feel jeopardized and what kind of information would tend to reassure her. She will also have a better idea of what she would be likely to do if she were to receive information that indicated a problem with the baby's health or development. Would her beliefs and her emotions compel her to carry the child to term anyway? Or does she feel unable or unwilling to cope with a high-need child? Knowing the answers to such questions will go a long way toward helping her decide what types, if any, of prenatal testing she feels are appropriate for her.

A woman who knows her options will be well acquainted, through reading and discussions with her obstetrician or midwife (and perhaps with a genetics counselor) not only with the ramifications of her particular family's health history, but with exactly what each test could, and could not, tell her. She will also be cognizant of any physiological risks associated with any test she is considering and of the percentage of erroneous results that each test may yield. This knowledge too will go a long way toward helping her make up her mind.

Armed with her knowledge of herself and of the medical pros and cons of each prenatal test, she should be able to resist anyone who tries to coerce her into doing the opposite of what she wants to do. Ideally, no one could talk her out of tests she feels are beneficial, nor could they scare or shame her into having tests she feels are inappropriate given her circumstances, her values, and her sensibilities.

A caveat, however. The system does not always function in an ideal manner. The propensity of obstetricians to lobby on behalf of the tests to their pregnant patients is strong. And it is probably not so much because they are wont to practice defensive medicine out of fear of malpractice suits, as is often suggested, as it is out of a technological bias instilled during their education.

As Perri Klass recounted, one of the phenomena that marked her tenure as a pregnant medical student was the inordinate number of fellow students who fussed over her solicitously, asking not how she was feeling but what sort of tests she'd undergone. "I cannot count the number of times I was asked whether I had had amniocentesis," writes Klass. When she reminded her classmates she was under 35 (the overwhelming majority of amniocentesis is performed on the basis of a maternal age over 34) they "tended to look worried and muttered something about being sure."

Continues Klass: "The height of the ridiculous came when a young man in class asked me, 'Have you had all those genetic tests? Like for sickle-cell anemia?' " Klass pointed out that she was Caucasian (so was the young man) and therefore not considered a potential carrier of this trait. " 'Yeah, I know,' " he said, " 'but if there's even a one in a million chance.' "[7]

It is easy to see how any mother-to-be, perhaps dubious about certain kinds of testing but concerned most of all with doing what's best for her child, might be tempted to let such a seed implant in her mind and blossom into full-fledged acceptance of any and all tests a well-meaning practitioner wants to administer. But she would be doing what's best for all concerned if she remembers that she has the right to ask for a good reason to undergo any procedure. Then it's finally up to her to say yes or no.

Ultimately, this sort of informed choice is the key to ensuring a reasonable amount of psychological comfort as well as physical well-being within the system.

❖ AN EXPECTANT MOTHER'S PRIVILEGES
AND PREROGATIVES

You're entitled to a supportive practitioner. You deserve to work with someone whose manner makes you feel comfortable and whose philosophy of prenatal care and childbirth is in keeping with your own. The more women make it clear that a feeling of support is one of the things they require and expect, the more this will gradually become the norm. We are, after all, medical *consumers*.

If a switch is in order, make it. If you have begun your prenatal care with someone whose attitudes make you feel uncomfortable (or in whom you do not have confidence for any reason), don't be afraid to make a change. You may well have some bureaucratic rigmarole to handle with your insurance carrier (for your financial well-being, it's important to let them know ahead of time and understand their policies), but paperwork in and of itself should not be enough of a deterrent to keep you in an unhappy situation. Before you commit to a new situation, make sure any practitioner you are considering knows why you were dissatisfied with the previous one. And, if you're so inclined, do the practitioner you're leaving a favor and explain diplomatically why his or her care was not right for you.

Information is critical; knowledge is power. Ask lots of questions, read, discuss, seek second opinions where you deem necessary. Learn what technology has to offer as well as what it does not offer. In short, get educated about the business of prenatal care and childbirth. During this process you may find that you simply feel better about the choice you were inclined to make in the first place. Or you may find that you alter your entire belief system. (For example, you may discover that your fear of labor is more a fear of hospitals and standard childbirth interventions than of the birth process itself and decide to do something non-mainstream.) Either way, you will never get what you want unless you're certain you know what you want—and that involves understanding the options.

You don't have to prove anything to anyone. The type of birth experience you elect to pursue really has nothing whatsoever to do with how politically correct a person you are, and even less to do with how good a mother you'll be. It has only to do with the personal informed choices of you and your husband. So beware those who proselytize for one sort of birth experience over another and who try to make you feel guilty when you don't see things their way. You can thank them politely for sharing their point of view and share your own view as well. But where dialogue serves, contentious debate does a disservice. Childbirth choices ought not present a forum for one-upmanship.

Make yourself understood. Be a conscientious communicator. Clearly express your wishes to those who will be involved in your prenatal care and in your baby's birth. Needless to say, it's best not to present yourself as combative or disrespectful. You want to set an example by your demeanor of how you would like your caregivers to respond to you.

A note to the "high risk" expectant mother: If your pregnancy has been defined as a "high risk" one, you may have the idea that you have no choices, or relatively few choices, as to how your prenatal care and childbirth experience will be conducted. But that is not so. Within the parameters of what is medically necessary, you may still find certain options are open to you. And certainly, like all pregnant women, it is your prerogative to work with a practitioner who is sensitive to your emotional circumstances as well as your physiological condition. Naturally, you will want to do all you can to assure a happy, healthy outcome for you and your new baby. That is why in your case it is especially essential to be informed. But do not presume you are powerless to influence the course of events.

By the way, in the Netherlands, where the prenatal and postpartum care of women is applauded by many for recognizing and honoring the human element, pregnancies are designated not as "low risk" and "high risk" but as "first line" (those likely to be uncomplicated) and "second line" (those requiring closer monitoring).[8] Conceptualizing your own pregnancy as "second line" might provide helpful to you, since the very phrase "high risk" can engender anxiety, make one feel at the mercy of the medical profession, and create a reluctance to ask questions and to participate in decision-making.

It can also make you feel your body is less wonderful and amazing than it actually is. What a shame that would be. For all pregnant bodies are marvels. Though, as we shall next see, they may take some getting used to.

4 *The Body Pregnant*

i'm 99% body. my brain has dissolved into
headaches tears confusion
my navel sticks out/eye of cyclops
my life for an apple fritter

—WANDA COLMAN
"Giving Birth"

Just over four months pregnant, and just over five pounds heavier, all around the tummy, I returned to my health club after a summer membership hiatus. I was determined to keep up an exercise regime that would guard against superfluous flabbiness during the remaining months of my baby's gestation. All summer I'd jogged, albeit more slowly than in previous summers, around the dirt path of the Central Park reservoir. Now, it was time for some cold weather routines—the familiar treadmills and Stairmasters.

Because I'd been an avid aerobics devotee for such a long time, I had my widwife's blessing to proceed. I also had a new leotard, freshly ordered from a maternity catalogue, which boasted a comfortable and practical wide support waistband. All I was lacking was the quintessential yuk-yuk pregnancy T-shirt, the one where a big red arrow points toward the belly and a caption announces: I'M NOT FAT, I'M PREGNANT.

Hey, this was no laughing matter. At this stage of the pregnancy, showing just a little bit, I harbored a mortal fear that all the specimens of perfect muscle tone who were huffing and puffing around me would size me up incorrectly and assume I'd spent my summer vacation at Ben and Jerry's.

Then, of course, I felt ashamed of myself. I should be proud of my changing body, right? And, in a way, I truly was. After all, it was a natural, beautiful thing. So what if I had been conditioned all my life by the "culture of slimness" and now faced the prospect of putting on pound after relentless pound? So what if I had no way of knowing for certain when, or if, I'd ever fit easily into my pre-pregnancy Calvins again? And so what if there were times I was so full of gas and water I felt like a public utility?

So, nothing. It was all fine. All worth it, no question. For what is vanity compared to the glories of motherhood?

Besides, there was plenty to distract me from obsessing on the shape of my body. Like trying to figure out why maternity clothes seemed to be designed by Mother Goose. And trying to find something—anything—to wear in these awkward in-between months when "real" clothes were too tight and full maternity regalia was still out of the question. And when I wasn't busy wondering what I should sport on my body, I was busy keeping tabs on what I put in it. The list of "no-no's" was long (good-bye apple pie, farewell Zinfandel), and the list of mineral-laden "must haves" was daunting.

I had to admit I was actually beginning to understand where mothers copped their martyr attitudes. I sent up a quick prayer that I would never actually say to my child words to the effect of, "I carried you for nine months, got stretch marks and gave up Mars Bars, and now you won't clean up your room!" Yet I could admit to myself that at some point in the not-so-distant future I might feel ever so slightly tempted to pull such a weapon out of my maternal arsenal.

Anyway for now, it was back to the treadmill. . . .

Expansion

The list of minor aches or ailments that might, at least from time to time, afflict an expectant mother is long. It includes sore and swollen feet, puffy ankles, back pain, tender joints, varicose veins, and sinus congestion. Add to this another list of irksome bodily generated inconveniences, for example, an urge to urinate only slightly less pressing than the urge to breathe, and a propensity to feel like one is being heated by one's own portable furnace. Add to this a list of assaults to one's vanity, for example, the moratorium one must declare on permanent waves and hair coloring, and one begins to understand why many women have mixed feelings about their bodies and their physical appearance during pregnancy.

But in our society there is one particular and unavoidable element of pregnancy that even the most sanguine of women may find disturbing. Given our cultural obsession with slimness, no one will be surprised to learn that this troublesome element is none other than the ubiquitous weight gain.

Nowadays the recommended weight gain for pregnant women is between 20 and 30 pounds. Anything less, it is warned, is insufficient to assure adequate infant size and good health. But even if it weren't recommended, I daresay many women would achieve comparable girth. For an expectant mother's appetite, usually beginning in the second trimester, can be a remarkable thing to behold.

All in all, significant weight gain in pregnancy is both a desirable and natural phenomenon. And if an objective observer completely unfamiliar with our cultural biases dropped in from, say, Pluto, he or she would probably have a hard time understanding why this aspect of pregnancy causes many women concern and some women outright misery. Yet anyone who inhabits the late twentieth-century Western world of planet Earth would understand.

For the whole of a woman's pre-pregnancy existence she is, both overtly and subtly, given one message in a thousand ways: Thin is good, gaining weight is bad. To complicate things, this is translated by far too many of us as: When you're thin *you* are good, when you gain weight *you* are bad. Self-esteem and weight issues are, alas, often so enmeshed that it is difficult indeed for one's psyche to break the problematical connection between them, even when a compelling reason presents itself.

Hence the expectant mother's dread of stepping on the scale. And the anxious queries she makes of other pregnant women ("How much have *you* gained so far?"). And the fear that what pounds go on won't come off. Hence the sense that the body is out of control, beyond reasoning with, off on a subversive tangent.

For women who have always perceived themselves as having a "weight problem" pregnancy-related gain can be especially difficult:

"Right before I got pregnant," said 24-year-old Jori, "I was at my thinnest ever and bought myself the best wardrobe I'd ever had. I knew I would have a child soon, and I guess I thought of it as my last hurrah. Then I got pregnant and gained weight, of course, and I felt myself going into mourning for that thin girl who I was so briefly and who I was sure I would never be again. Sometimes I would open my closet and just stare at my size six clothes. It was hard to imagine I'd ever worn them at all."

"I had always been a dieter," said 34-year-old Valerie. "To me, the longer I could go without eating, the more virtuous I felt. So I promptly had an identity crisis when I hit my second trimester and felt like eating constantly. I considered this appetite a real problem, but I'd get on the scale at my obstetrician's office and the nurse would say, "Good girl" when I'd gained several pounds and shake her head in disapproval when I seemed to be plateauing for a while. I kept thinking how surreal it all seemed."

Even women who generally felt comfortable with their weight and their relationship to their bodies before can have body image problems during pregnancy, especially when the pounds first start to add up:

"I read somewhere," said 31-year-old Jennifer, "that if the baby's growth accelerated at the rate it was going during the fourth month of pregnancy a baby would come out weighing fourteen *tons*. It was a funny bit of trivia, but it ended up giving me a pretty wild nightmare. I dreamed I became enormous, big as a house. I kept asking, when is this baby coming out already, so I can trim down? A doctor came in and said, 'Congratulations, you've had a baby elephant.' And the worst part was, I was still as big as a house!"

And even women who feel they can pretty well tolerate the idea of gaining around 30 pounds for their babies' sake can encounter problems when they encounter the opinions of others. A teasing husband, no matter how well-meaning and loving his quips, can send an expectant mother into paroxysms of self-doubt. As for a pregnant woman's own mother, when it comes to matters of weight, her input can carry a good deal of it. This is unfortunate, because most of our mothers gave birth during an era when women were strongly cautioned against gaining more than 15 pounds during pregnancy. Genuinely alarmed that their daughters are ballooning into the danger zone, their evaluations can be harsh, to say the least. ("Oh, my dear," said one mother on visiting her pregnant daughter, "it's triplets for certain." It was not triplets, nor twins for that matter. Indeed her daughter gained the ideal "textbook" amount of weight for a healthy mother of one, carrying in her second trimester.)

Of course, no matter what her mother or husband or even what she may think of it, if all is proceeding normally, the weight gain of an expectant mother will continue as her baby grows and thrives. Were this an "ordinary" weight gain, the woman might have some wardrobe recourse. But this is one situation where clothes present even further conundrums.

"As soon as my jeans got too tight, I went into a panic," recalled 30-year-old Jeannine. "I swore I'd never wear actual maternity clothes so I went out and got a whole bunch of things with elastic waistbands. Guess what? I rapidly learned the limits of elasticity."

"I wanted to put off maternity clothing purchases for as long as possible," said 38-year-old Patti, "but I found out most maternity stores tend to stock outfits for the coming season rather than the current one, just like regular clothing stores. I knew I'd have to buy summer clothes in spring, especially since there were a couple of formal affairs I'd have to attend late in my pregnancy. I went to try things on and felt ridiculous. I was swimming in the clothes. I couldn't ever picture being so large. When they gave me a 'pregnancy pillow' to fill me out I felt even more ridiculous. I thought, 'You look just like a little girl trying to play dress up.' "

When it comes to issues of self-image, one of the most difficult times for the expectant mother in this country seems to be the early to middle second trimester—otherwise known as The Great Wardrobe Limbo. It is a period when nothing looks or fits quite right and many women are fearful that the world at large is perceiving them not as blossoming mothers-to-be but rather as insatiable french fry aficionados.

In Japan, a woman who is five months pregnant goes through a ritual where she is fitted with a *hara obi*, a wide abdominal sash.[1] Wearing this helps her acknowledge her condition to herself—and to everyone else. Here, we have no such affirmative ritual. Stretched-out leggings and oversized T-shirts are the traditional garments of limbo, and their purpose is not to proclaim but to camouflage.

Thankfully, however, the limbo period does not go on forever and camouflage doesn't work forever. Before one knows it, there is simply no mistaking the fact that one is with child, rather than simply with bloat. And, though women in the early limbo phase may have a hard time believing it, things generally improve at that "point of no return."

Once a woman is visibly, undeniably in the midst of pregnancy she may have an easier time accepting her new spherical voluptuousness. Now, at least, even casual observers (all but the most obtuse) will comprehend what's really going on. Now she can eat heartily without seeming unseemly. Now her maternity clothes, though perhaps too frilly and doll-like for her taste, at least seem to serve a bona fide purpose.

Slowly but surely, she may begin to enjoy aspects of her changing appearance. In some cases, she may even flaunt it, whether in clothing or out of it.

Vanity's Fair

In August, 1991, actress Demi Moore, extremely pregnant with her second daughter, caused a stir when she appeared in an

Annie Lebovitz photo on the cover of *Vanity Fair* wearing nothing but diamonds. As the magazine reported a year later, the shot provoked "heated debate."[2]

The controversy, centering on the appropriateness of presenting a pregnant woman in an eroticized manner, was in a way peculiar. For century after century in culture upon culture, large-breasted, big-bellied, pregnant women were celebrated by artists and craftspeople, re-created in countless carvings and statues. As the quintessence of yin, the feminine principle, the pregnant form was revered. There was no symbol which more clearly denoted fertility, sensuality, and the fruits of passion.

But in our society, some were offended, making a case that such a photograph betrayed, of all things, family values. Even pregnant women themselves were divided, but not, for the most part, on moral grounds. (Family values, indeed!)

The real issue among those I spoke with seemed to center on to what degree they could personally relate to the actress's pregnant-and-proud stance. Some found that the image of a sexy pregnant woman validated a delightfully mischievous, titillating feeling they had been harboring deep down inside that pregnancy had rendered them sexier than ever. As one woman said:

> "It took me a while to get used to it, but I never felt so exquisitely sexy as now. Being pregnant is the most erotically charged time in my life. I feel at the peak of my female powers, alluring, seductive, and earthy."

But some said, whoa. Sexy and pregnant? Fetching and pregnant? Even among expectant mothers who were gradually growing more comfortable with their evolving shapes, many felt playing the temptress and the goddess was quite the leap. (As we'll see in a later chapter, there are many factors in addition to body image which affect a woman's level of sexual desire during pregnancy.)

Still, though they may have never entertained the notion, let alone had the opportunity, of displaying their bodies Demi-style for the masses, many expressed the wish to experience more of this yin winsomeness in their private lives. As one mother-to-be put it, "I wish I could feel half that frisky."

Babying Oneself

If you do wish to feel kindlier toward and prouder of your pregnant body, consider beginning a regime that will assist you in this process as your pregnancy progresses. For when carrying a baby, you need to baby yourself on a physical level.

Throughout much of history in most parts of the world, the pregnant woman was encouraged to treat her body reverently and tend it lovingly. She practiced yoga or other forms of calming and balancing movement. She was massaged and rubbed with oils. And the regular exercise which was necessarily part of her life was not discouraged so long as it was moderate.

Then, in seventeenth- and eighteenth-century Europe, things changed. Routine pregnancy came to be viewed as a state of unwellness and expectant mothers were cautioned against any number of "dangerous practices" from dancing (considered the height of recklessness) to standing in the breeze (both north and south winds were said to bring about the loss of babies) to sitting with their legs crossed (which supposedly led to deformed children and lengthened labor). Engaging in any circular motion, including the suspiciously dervishlike endeavors of grinding coffee and unwinding balls of wool, was forbidden on the grounds the umbilical cord would twist itself around the infant.[3]

What's more, for reasons that remain elusive, various medical texts also warned that a pregnant woman who spent too much time doing her hair was chancing a miscarriage. Apparently, an expectant mother's behavior was considered suspect and hazardous if she did pretty much *anything* to make herself feel good.

Now, fortunately, everything old is new again. Gone are the days when pregnant women were counseled to live in fear of ruinous north winds and perilous balls of wool. Indeed, as social psychologist Carol Tavris has noted, more and more contemporary women "have rejected the notion that to be pregnant is to be sick."[4]

Pregnant women today, after thanking their lucky stars that they did not incarnate in early modern Europe, can take a lesson from the era which predated that period. They can treat their bodies with the respect they deserve. What's more, they can have a good time doing so.

Being massaged, for example, is an excellent way to ease aching joints and muscle tension induced by carrying extra weight. It is an excellent natural antidote to stress (especially useful when any chemical antidotes are strictly off limits). Equally important, it makes one feel soothed and cared for. In the hands of a professional who has experience with maternity massage, a woman can anticipate a blissful interlude. And if a professional is out of range, financially or geographically, husbands are often happy to play masseur—though they should be reminded to do so *gently*. (From my fourth month on my husband dutifully rubbed cocoa butter on my stretching skin every night before bed. Not only did it feel wonderful, but it worked as a stretch mark preventative.)

As for exercise, if one's midwife or doctor agrees that it is beneficial (they almost surely will if a pregnancy is routine), there is no better tonic for the pregnant woman who is feeling blue about her physical self. Exercise is an energizer and an overall mood enhancer. Many believe it is a way of increasing flexibility and stamina needed for childbirth. And it is certainly a way of increasing self-esteem. Many women commented to me that they felt immeasurably better about their changing bodies once they resolved to keep active. And happily, there are more opportunities to do so than ever. Prenatal exercise classes are proliferating and exercise videos for mothers-to-be show signs of becoming a growth industry. (Even as this paragraph is being written, Rachel Hunter, supermodel and wife of Rod Stewart, is said to be having a video—and a baby—in the making.)

As an addition to aerobic and toning exercise, many women very much enjoy prenatal yoga. It helps with physical balance and with psychic balance as well. In fact, because of its emphasis on harmonizing body and mind, it is an ideal pursuit for the pregnant woman who wants to stop thinking of her body as an adversary. (See Suggestions for Further Reading at the back of this book for references on prenatal yoga and exercise.)

Naturally enough, accommodations must be made. When it comes to exercise, one can't expect to maintain the level of agility one had before. Nor is this a good time to take up a new sport. It's essential to discuss with one's practitioner the type and amount of activity that one plans to engage in—and to know when to quit. For competitive types, it's important to refrain from comparing one's performance with that of nonpregnant women who are, so to speak, playing in a different league. (To avoid this potential self-esteem pitfall, some prefer taking a prenatal exercise class with other pregnant women to trying to keep up with former aerobics compatriots.)

Even yoga must be done amidst certain constraints. A pregnant woman should not expect, for example, to spend time standing on her head or doing anything too exotic or extreme. As for massage, its techniques and level of intensity must take the baby into account. There are certain things, such as avoiding the abdominal area in the first trimester, that one's practitioner ought to be able to clarify.

But apart from observing such sensible caveats, a woman in the midst of a routine pregnancy may reap the many benefits of babying herself in these ways—including not only a sprier body, but a more confident and spirited mind-set, greater satisfaction with her appearance, and greater overall self-regard.

In the bargain, by routinely babying yourself in these healthful ways, you may find it easier to abandon some of the old routines which pregnancy mandated you forfeit—such as the glass of wine each evening or full jug of morning coffee. One doesn't want to perpetuate such habits during pregnancy for the obvious reason that they can be harmful to the baby. Also, indulging in them can contribute to yet another psychological dilemma, namely . . .

The Guilts

What a woman puts on her outer body—clothing, makeup, extra weight—is, like it or not, for all the world to see. But what she puts inside her body is generally considered a private matter. Until she becomes pregnant, that is. Then this too becomes a topic for public discussion.

By the time a woman is into her second trimester, she most likely has a daily "do and don't" litany going round in her head virtually all the time. The *dos* go: Eat your greens, take your vitamins, drink two quarts of water, eat a yellow vegetable, have lots of fiber, meet your calcium and protein quotas. Don't forget those foods high in iron, like sardines and blackstrap molasses. The *don'ts* go: Watch out for caffeine (even in chocolate), forget about alcohol, easy on the salt, no fatty foods at the evening meal, ix-nay on the junk food, steer clear of fish with a high mercury content, throw out the saccharin. Et cetera, et cetera.

Such advice is often given by doctors and midwives, which is as it ought to be. But it is also frequently reiterated by well-meaning husbands, friends, and relations, many of whom suddenly appoint themselves the expectant mother's newly appointed nutritionist *and* conscience all rolled into one. ("That has *white sugar* in it," they can sometimes be heard to gasp, making the nibbler of a lone Oreo feel like she has been chain-smoking unfiltered Camels.) Such secondhand editorializing, many expectant mothers feel, is *not* as it ought to be. Many consider it patronizing and intrusive.

To the chagrin of pregnant women, even waiters have been known to get in on the act, serving up a side dish of guilt to a mother-to-be who decides to dabble publicly in a weensy special occasion cheat. As one mother-to-be recalled:

> "I was visibly pregnant and lunching with an old friend who was in from out of town. It was the middle of a hectic day. When it came time for dessert my companion asked for espresso, for which this café was well known, and I said I'd have one too. The waiter said, 'Decaf, right?' I said, 'No, regular.' He stared at me for a second and whispered, 'Let me bring you some nice herb tea.' I hate herb tea. I knew one espresso wasn't going to produce dire consequences. So I stuck to my guns. But I didn't enjoy my coffee after that. I felt like I'd been branded with a scarlet C, for caffeine."

Dos and don'ts may even be reiterated by one's insurance company, which has financial as well as humanitarian motives for facilitating a healthy pregnancy. There's nothing inherently wrong with some precautionary pamphlets, but some women consider their proliferation a bit of an overkill.

> "My health insurance carrier sent a bulky packet of ominous warnings with no less than five brochures warning against alcohol, tobacco, and drug use during pregnancy. One I would have appreciated, but five? Was I on some kind of list? Had someone been watching me when I was in college?"

Not too surprisingly, many expectant mothers take umbrage at this sort of thing. The fact that they are charged with the responsibility and privilege of ushering life into the world is hardly lost on the vast majority of mothers-to-be. Do they also need the constant supervision of self-appointed pregnancy police?

For as long as women have been getting pregnant, each culture has had its recommendations of what women should and shouldn't ingest while carrying a baby. Some of those recommendations and prohibitions have withstood the test of time. (Many tribal cultures, for instance, discouraged sweets and fats in excess as well as very salty food.) Others seem laughable when we look back on them. (In eighteenth-century Europe, the medical profession warned against such foodstuffs as hazelnuts and hard-boiled eggs.)[5] But in all of this there is one constant: It is rare for a pregnant woman to encounter anyone who does not have a pointer or two on the subject of what she ought to eat and what she ought to avoid.

What to do?

Once again, information is the expectant mother's best friend. Reading some information on pregnancy nutrition and asking questions of your practitioner will arm you with the information you need to make wise decisions. It will also allow you to make reasonable choices as to which items are absolutely verboten and which can be considered special, occasional dalliances. Beyond that, common sense goes a long way in making such discriminations, though many people try to make the expectant mother think otherwise.

It does not require a doctorate to figure out that one piece of pizza with anchovies isn't going to rocket the blood pressure of a person whose blood pressure is consistently normal. Yet I have a friend who deprived herself of this, her favorite delicacy, for months out of fear that the extra sodium would send her straight into a state of toxemia. When she finally could stand it no longer, she ate the anchovies and washed them down with a liter of guilty tears.

Her behavior was not atypical, for when it comes to little cheats, the guilt of a mother-to-be is often disproportionate to her transgression. It is partly because she cares so much about her baby. But it is also partly because the pregnancy police, well-meaning though they may be, have implanted in her psyche the notion that she is perhaps a tad inadequate in fulfilling her maternal duties.

You're *most* adequate and should remember that. Your pregnant body is a wondrous thing. It is working round the clock to do its job and do it well. It is growing a baby, complete with limbs, heart, and brain. Following an ancient blueprint, it is creating the world all over again, *in a way no other particular body can duplicate.*

Of course, it needs special attention. But bestowing that attention upon it can be, if one lets it, much more of a pleasure than a chore.

❖ AN EXPECTANT MOTHER'S PRIVILEGES AND PREROGATIVES

Give yourself permission to eat when you are hungry. If you are like many women, the very natural act of taking nourishment may long have engendered mixed feelings in you. Though you may have longed to eat with gusto, perhaps you've had the idea that to do so would not only be "bad" for you but would be frowned upon by society. Now, sing hallelujah. It's time to give yourself permission to eat and eat hearty when your appetite summons you. You have to do it in order to keep up your strength and grow a healthy baby. So you might as well enjoy it. Consider your pregnancy interlude a blessed hiatus from food-related remorse. (Having said this, I hasten to add that if you find yourself eating not out of hunger but in order to dull an emotion such as anxiety or sadness, choose to have the emotion instead of the food. Emotional overeating is a bad habit to get into, and a difficult one to break, pregnant or not.)

Take control of your "weigh-ins." One of the potential stress points of any prenatal exam is the moment when the nurse says cheerfully, "Okay, let's step up on that scale." (The word *let's*, of course, is a purely rhetorical device.) In order to monitor the pregnancy, most practitioners will want to check to make sure that you are gaining a sufficient amount of weight. But that doesn't mean you have to listen to a running commentary about your gain, provided it's within the realm of acceptable.

In some birthing clinics, women are charged with the responsibility of weighing themselves and recording their weight on their charts sans audience. I have known several women who have broken tradition in obstetrical offices and requested to do the same, as well as some mothers-to-be who preferred to have the nurses silently weigh them while they stared into space, choosing to ignore the scales' precise measurement.

A number on a scale is just that, a number. And most of it reflects things like the weight of the baby, the placenta, and extra body fluids. But if hearing a number tends to make you upset (perhaps even to the point where it may cause you to try to cut back on needed nutrients) try to arrange with your practitioner a way to alleviate your anxiety.

Move it! (And have it moved for you.) Try to take advantage of the burgeoning opportunities for expectant mothers to remain active. Check your area for offerings in pregnancy exercise, dance, and yoga classes. And check for masseuses skilled in working with pregnant women. Along with the many benefits already mentioned, this will offer you more opportunities to network with other expectant mothers and to learn more about what's happening to your amazing body.

If you feel like it, flaunt it. Some women don't feel sexy at all during pregnancy, others feel sexier than ever. Many fall in the middle of the spectrum but feel especially sexy some of the time (maybe when their husbands compliment them, maybe when they've had a good exercise session, maybe when their estrogen is especially frisky). If you do feel like being a little racy, enjoy yourself in whatever way feels appropriate for you. You might want to turn down the lights and put on some romantic music when you ask your husband to massage your stretching tummy, or suggest a warm bath for two (well, three actually). Even those Mother Goose maternity clothes can be made more alluring with a little alteration and imagination. One can always raise a hemline, bare a shoulder, and accessorize with flair. (I had a friend who, unable to find anything remotely glamorous to wear to a wedding while she was pregnant, bought a simple A-line swing dress, shortened it, replaced its plain buttons with elegant faux pearl and rhinestone ones, left the top few open, and enjoyed the compliments she got from everyone around.)

Keep the time frame in perspective. Though it may be hard to believe when you first start to bulge, the next few months of your pregnancy will probably find you growing more comfortable with your evolving shape and size. But even if you never quite get used to it, remember that in the great scheme of things this only lasts a short while. During the relatively brief period of pregnancy, the body is a vehicle for new life, and each choice you make for your body directly impacts another's body. You need to surrender to that truth, and in surrendering liberate yourself from undue obsessions. Once this time is passed, you can, after a reasonable recuperation period, run ultra-marathons, diet on grapefruit and crackers, or stand on your head for hours on end if any of that makes you happy.

(On the other hand, who knows? Maybe pregnancy will rid you of such extreme urges forevermore. Some women report that after bearing their children they feel much more at ease with their bodies overall, and no longer feel the need to focus on every half pound fluctuation the way they might have before.)

Use your body as a source of information. The more you respect your body, the more you'll feel in harmony with it, and the more receptive you will be to its cues. On some level, your body knows exactly what to do to keep healthy during the pregnancy. It knows when you need to slow down and rest. It knows when you need to eat more or drink more liquids. Pay attention and it will tell you these things. And when it tells you, take it seriously.

The body has much work to occupy it now and its demands should be honored. But the mind has much to occupy it as well, and even now it is working overtime ruminating on just who this baby of yours will turn out to be. And that is the subject of the next chapter.

5 The Imaginary Baby

Of all passing notions, that of a human being for a child is perhaps the purest in the abstract, and the most complicated in reality.

—LOUISE ERDRICH
"A Woman's Work"

In my fifth month of pregnancy I not only felt good, but even began to believe I looked good. My queasiness and my sense of "lumpiness" was behind me, and the unwieldiness of late pregnancy lay in the distant future. True to cliché, people said I "glowed," and I confess I felt a bit luminescent. I had the vague notion that something momentous was about to happen, and one day it did. I was sitting at my desk transcribing some notes when I felt a strange flutter. My baby began, ever so gently, to soft-shoe his way across my abdomen.

Up until that moment, my pregnancy had been mostly a time of self-preoccupation, which is not uncommon and certainly not unwarranted. Now I became entranced with visions of my fellow traveler, my "womb-mate." Who was this tapping at me from the inside? What was he up to?

Several times in past months I'd made a particular Freudian slip, referring to my uterus as my "universe." Now I found I liked to think of my baby as that vast firmament's sole inhabitant, drifting in blissful quietude, free of desire and

*of the constraints of time. What would he be like, I won-
dered. (I said him, even then, not because any test had indicated gender, but because I strongly sensed a yang energy, a
masculine presence.) And what would he think of me?*

*In many Eastern religions there's an intriguing and I think
comforting concept which says that souls coming into the
world actually choose their parents in order to play out their
karma, or destiny, and learn the lessons they must learn in
this one of many lifetimes. But what sort of incoming soul
might choose me as its mother—and why?*

*Like nearly all mothers-to-be, I began to evaluate my ca-
pacity for nurturing, and probably like most, I found myself
wanting. In my most insecure moments I obsessed: Was I too
selfish to be a mother? Too absorbed in my own affairs? Too
controlling? Too set in my ways? But, if so, why had some
sentient soul selected me? Perhaps he hadn't. Perhaps it was
all random, after all. Maybe this unsuspecting baby had no
idea what he was in for. Maybe he had no idea that his mother
still hadn't been able to make a simple decision about disposable versus cloth diapers, let alone figure out whatever else
was required of her.*

*In any case, whether his showing up was premeditated or
random, this child would have his own destiny to fulfill, and
in that destiny I would play a crucial role. Would we be a
good match, this "imaginary baby" and I? Would we get
along, enjoy each other's company? I never questioned
whether we would love each other. In fact there were moments, as I felt his increasingly ambitious somersaults, when
I was overcome with tender emotions for this perfect
stranger. But as my pregnancy progressed I worried more and
more about whether we would like each other, whether we
would be as good a fit after birth as before. . . .*

Womb-Mates

Sometime around the eighteenth to twentieth week of pregnancy, perhaps a bit sooner if this is a second or subsequent

child, a woman begins to notice little flickers of movement inside her. At first, especially for a first-time mother, there may be some confusion about what is going on. She's likely been asked already if she has felt the baby moving, and she's been impatiently and eagerly anticipating it. But when it actually occurs she may be surprised to experience a sensation far more gentle and subtle than she was prepared for. For the most part, the era of super-animated kicking and punching (the kind you can actually see through your sweater) lies a little in the future. The first tangible signs of the baby's activity can feel suspiciously like tiny gas bubbles to some, until the eventual revelation dawns that *this is it*, the real thing.

Certainly by now, bulging tummies have contributed to the expectant mother's dawning revelation that, yes, there's an actual flesh and bone baby in there. So have sonograms, if they have been administered. (As one woman, recounting her reactions to ultrasound, wrote in *The New Yorker*: "The picture shocked me . . . thrilled me for the extension of my powers, surprised me by its concrete actuality . . ."[1]) Still, nothing drives the point of the viability of one's child as having it *do* something which can be tangibly perceived.

Once a mother-to-be figures out what the bubbly sensations inside her actually signify, her response can be impassioned. From that moment on, the emotional tone of the pregnancy can alter dramatically. Instead of feeling like mothers-to-be, many pregnant women begin to feel like they too are becoming the real thing—genuine, card-carrying mothers:

> "Before I felt the baby move," said 25-year-old Janice, "I thought of the pregnancy as something I was doing. Now I thought of it as something I was helping with. I was helping this baby be born. It had a purpose, a life of its own, and I was helping it fulfill that purpose."

In addition to feeling more of an emotional connection with her child as it wiggles and stretches, a woman may experience a palpable sense of relief regarding matters physiological.

> "I had several tests before I felt the baby, and they all indicated things were fine," said 38-year-old Randy. "But that didn't do it

for me. I never truly felt secure about the baby's well-being. It took the baby's moving for me to feel she was really okay. Now, the movement was something I began to look forward to every day."

And some women, understandably enough, consider the awesome event of the baby's early bustling to be a spiritual watershed, whether this is a first pregnancy or a later one:

"I remember this very particular moment one night when I felt my first daughter move," recalled 31-year-old Katrine. "I sat up in bed and started to cry. I woke up my husband and said, 'Oh God, *someone is in here with me.'* I was overwhelmed, amazed, and scared. It was as though I could feel her soul. A couple of years later, a similar thing happened with my son. I could feel his very, very strong spirit inside me. It just knocked me out."

In all these instances, a new dimension has been added to the pregnancy, and this is consciously reflected. An expectant mother begins to talk about the things her baby is doing and to speculate about its characteristics.

Often mothers-to-be experience strong hunches where their babies are concerned. No doubt some of these could represent "wishful thinking," for all of us have some preconceived notions about the kinds of children we would, ideally, like to enlist in our family ranks. But some premonitions do turn out to be uncannily accurate.

We have probably all met women who say they "just knew" they were pregnant virtually from the moment of conception. Similar intuitive leaps may come upon a woman at any time during her baby's gestation. I talked with women whose prenatal predictions about everything from their babies' appearance ("He'll be bald with his father's dimple." "She'll have a head full of black hair and her grandma's big feet.") to character traits ("This one will be a real charmer, the life of the party.") and even talents ("This one is musical, like his dad. I can tell he feels happy when music is playing.") were, quite remarkably, borne out. And any number of women will tell you that they needed no medically sanctioned tests to tell them whether their little tenants were boys or girls.

Not all of this remarkable intuitive process is easily explain-
able, and one cannot help but surmise that there is a deep con-
nectedness between a childbearing woman and her growing
baby that defies rational cause-and-effect explanation and takes
us into another realm altogether. On the other hand, at least
some sorts of so-called hunches may have to do with simply
paying attention.

The baby, through its level and nature of activity, patterns of
movement, and times of locomotion and quietude, may indeed
be offering the observant woman clues about its nature and its
habits. Many women swear that their babies maintained the
same schedule after birth as they seemed to be keeping before.
Others firmly believe that they could tell during pregnancy
which of their children would be more dynamic and which more
mellow by the nature of their intrauterine movements.

From a combination of all their thoughts, fantasies, and
"hunches" (whether, in fact, they ultimately turn out accurate
or not), and observations, pregnant women build a conscious
set of expectations about their babies, which they carry through
the remainder of their pregnancies and which color their visions
of what life will be like once the babies have arrived. Their unconscious processes also reflect some of their deeper optimistic
or pessimistic expectations.

In their dream life expectant mothers process the sensation
of having an active passenger—one with a *personality*—on
board in any number of ways. Some dream of playing with and
caring for a happy, smiling child. Some dream of being unable
to comfort a crying child. Many dream of conversing with their
babies. Some imagine giving birth to a walking, talking child
who emerges from the womb with a full set of opinions about a
wide range of topics (not the least of which is what kind of a job
he or she thinks Mom is doing).

Symbols, of course, play a key role in dream life, and each
stage of pregnancy can represent certain aspects of the mother's
perceptions of her baby. According to a study conducted by San
Francisco's Neonatal and Obstetrical Research Laboratory,
among the most common dream objects appearing in an expectant mother's first trimester are worms and potted plants. Come

the second trimester, she dreams more frequently of cute, furry animals, such as kittens.[2] This would seem to be indicative not only of her sense that her child is becoming more "playful" and "alive" in the womb, but also of her greater degree of emotional involvement with her baby (kittens being more huggable than potted plants and more responsive than worms).

Not too surprisingly, women beginning to feel their babies move about also tend to report a high incidence of dreams centering on the theme of intruders. They envision people breaking into their homes (as, indeed, one soon will). Some even dream of encountering alien beings. This is not startling either, considering they are literally in the midst of a "space" invasion.

In the light of day, the intrusion dreams which may have seemed so vivid and unsettling during the night tend to pale and recede in intensity. Nevertheless, their significance cannot be discounted. The expectant mother's psyche is trying to process the incredible truth that an unknown being will shortly alter her life irrevocably.

But is this child so unknown? Or can she get to know it? And can she make *herself* known to her child in some way? If she could, she might feel less frightened. So the mother-to-be wonders—and hopes. Surely, there must be a means of communicating with a being that is *part* of her at that very instant. In her own way, perhaps ever so tentatively at first, she typically entertains the idea of making contact with her child.

A Womb With a View?

In his discourse on the *Duties of Mothers Toward their Children During Pregnancy,* Erasmus stated a belief that the qualities of babies' bodies and minds are developed in the womb. He suggested that mothers ought "not neglect to prepare and school them, even in this state, in honest Christian behavior."[3] If this sounds a little overambitous (or downright pompous), not to worry. It's unlikely that any such input would mean much to a womb-entrenched baby, who has neither frame of reference nor immediate practical use for ethical precepts anyhow. But that's not to say that certain types of input won't get through to a developing infant.

Those who study prenatal neurology and psychology have found evidence that, to some extent, babies in the womb can "see" and "hear." At four months, research has shown, a baby can perceive a bright light shining on its mother's stomach. At five months, the infant will react to loud sounds by laying its hands across its ears. It is even said that babies in the womb can discriminate between voices or between, say, pieces of music.

Indeed many parents swear they have observed their newborn babies after birth perking up at the sound of Mom or Dad's familiar voice, or at the sound of a concerto Mom played over and over again during gestation. Studies at Queens University in Northern Ireland and at the University of Carolina at Greensboro have backed up such anecdotal evidence, demonstrating that newborns preferred sounds to which they'd become acclimated before birth.[4]

This is all rather intriguing. As is the idea that babies in vivo even exhibit physiological signs associated with REM (rapid eye movement) dream sleep.[5] But, if their senses are operative and if they're capable of "dreaming," how much are babies in the womb capable of understanding?

No one is quite sure, though many expectant mothers certainly act as if significant comprehension on their children's behalf were a foregone conclusion. They instinctively talk to their developing infants, often by names they have already picked out for them or by affectionate nicknames. They coo and sing to them, often encouraging their spouses to do the same. Some play their favorite music for them, as a way of introducing them to the things they enjoy. Some tell the babies things about themselves and the homes that await them. Some even joke with their babies or pass the time making idle chitchat.

In the Netherlands, prenatal parent/child contact has been developed and structured into a discipline known as "haptonomy." Mothers- and fathers-to-be frequent classes where they are instructed in focusing on the baby in the uterus. Each parent practices hands-on stroking and caressing through the abdominal wall. They speak to the baby in a soothing fashion, and so on. Perryn Rowland, a childbirth educator and labor coach who visited the Netherlands while pregnant herself and who took haptonomy classes with her husband, describes the purpose of the classes as "promoting an enjoyable way of beginning the parent-child bonding process."

Exactly how much emotional benefit the baby gets out of such endeavors, be they structured, as in haptonomy, or more random, is still to a large extent a compelling mystery. Obviously, exposure to stimuli helps familiarize us with those stimuli, so it seems reasonable to assume that being born into a world where some things are, in some sense, already familiar may ameliorate certain stresses. Beyond that, most people tend to believe what they like.

Yet whatever your personal beliefs about how much comfort your womb-bound baby will take from receiving aural and tactile expressions of parental affection, it surely couldn't hurt to attempt to make such contact. Especially because many emotional benefits of attempted prenatal communication should accrue to you. Consciously attempting to make contact with one's baby is an act of intimacy in which one "rehearses" attempting to understand one's child and making oneself understood in turn. It can, by creating a sense of the familiar and the familial, at times help ease fears of the unknown and promote feelings of calm.

But do take note. I say *at times*, because, realistically speaking, no expectant mother will be calm all of the time, no matter how much she may wish it and no matter how much love for her baby she may manifest and express. Ironically, there will be times when the very fact that your imaginary baby is becoming much more real to you than before is itself a potential source of uneasiness. Not because you don't feel tenderly toward your child ("intruder" though he or she may be), but because you may not be feeling tenderly toward yourself. Because you may dread turning into the worst and scariest of all possible creatures you can envision right now: the quintessential "bad mother."

Self-Indictment

The term used to describe the sensation of the infant moving in the womb is *quickening*. In the first of its several dictionary definitions, to "quicken" literally means to animate or vivify. But it also means to accelerate, to hasten. This seems equally applicable to the expectant mother's circumstances. The baby's newly action-packed days and nights serve as a woman's reminder that she can't stay pregnant forever. Before much more time elapses there will be a new baby to tend.

If this is her first child, this emotional epiphany will probably leave a pregnant woman feeling somewhat unprepared and inadequate. But even if this is her second, third, or fourth child, she may well feel the same.

Any new child presents fresh challenges and brings significant stresses to the family unit. And most mothers-to-be, in their more insecure moments (often at 4 A.M. or so, just after their babies have awakened them by using their bladders as trampolines) contrive long lists of reasons why they are not up to tackling the job at hand, for example:

"*I'm too set in my ways.* This baby will disrupt all my routines, turn my life upside down. I'll feel way too impatient to have my life back the way it was before."

"*I'm too much of a perfectionist.* I will want this child to be brilliant, gorgeous, perfectly behaved, exceptional. I'll put too much pressure on him and turn into one of those pushy, overachiever mothers everybody loathes."

"*I'm too lazy.* A new baby will require constant attention. And I'll be up all hours. I'm really a sloth at heart, likely to be neglectful of his needs."

"*I'm too short-tempered.* The baby will fuss and I'll get mad. I hope I don't 'lose it' and turn into a shrew. Who knows how many thousands it will cost to pay for the child psychologist."

"*I'm overprotective.* I'll worry constantly and turn this child into a clingy bundle of nerves. He'll live at home until he's forty."

"*I'm too moody.* Sometimes I know I'm capable of being very kind and nurturing. Other times I'm just as irritable as can be. I'll be the Jekyll and Hyde of mothers."

"*I'm a pushover.* I have a hard time saying no. I think I'll do anything not to see my child unhappy. He'll end up running the house, no doubt, and grow up a sociopath."

"*I feel like a child myself.* When I was little I thought grown-ups knew everything. But now I still feel like I don't know much of anything. I'm not nearly as wise as a mother ought to be. How will someone be able to depend on me?"

In the wee hours women toss and turn, indicting themselves in advance for the "sins of the mothers" they are sure they will commit. If they already have children, they may tally up the "mistakes" they think they've made so far. And if they are mothering rookies, they may recall in exaggeratedly lurid detail each and every time they felt utterly befuddled when faced with a distraught or mischievous child who belonged to someone else. As one novice expectant mother recalled:

"I first announced to my family I was pregnant while I was visiting my family for Thanksgiving. Everyone was thrilled, but they also teased me a lot—asking if I was really ready for motherhood. One day, my brother and sister-in-law, who were also at our family gathering, asked if I would watch their two-year-old twin girls while they ran a quick errand. Everyone else was busy and I felt I had to agree, and besides I thought I needed the practice. They were no sooner out the door, though, when one of the twins began throwing up. As I bent over to tend to her, the other climbed on top of a chair, quick as a jackrabbit, and toppled over backwards.

"The girls both ended up fine, as it turned out. But by the time their parents returned I was a quivering wreck. I thought, 'That's it. I can never handle motherhood. Who am I kidding?' My husband had to calm me down over and over that night, reminding me that I wasn't going to be giving birth to two two-year-olds, that I would get to know and learn to handle our baby one step at a time."

Rather than chalking up her unsettling baby-sitting episode to a coincidence of mildly unfortunate events peppered by a dose of inexperience, this expectant mother quite typically imagined herself to be maternally incompetent. Like so many, she judged herself harshly before all the evidence was in. In a society where everyone seems only too happy to point the finger of wrongdoing at mothers on a regular basis, pregnant women seem only too happy to jump on the bandwagon.

But they usually don't take all the blame on themselves. In fact, while they are indicting themselves, they often name a co-conspirator. It is someone they believe may have committed worse offenses than even *they* are capable of. And they vow never to be like her. But they are afraid they might turn out just so.

Not Like My Mother!

Quickening, it turns out, has yet another dictionary definition. It can mean to provoke and arouse. This too is relevant to the pregnant woman in the sense that the baby's discernible movement in the womb, its subsequent enhanced "reality," and the woman's own looming task of mothering arouse in her many feelings about what it was like to *be* mothered. This can provoke some intense memories and, in turn, some powerful emotions, in the same way that the first trimester's sense of smell triggered memories both poignant and painful—but ultimately useful.

None of us was mothered perfectly, of course, for all of our mothers were human and hence imperfect. But many women feel their mothers' way of mothering was more imperfect than others. Sometimes they have genuine and serious grievances.

Sometimes they and their mothers were not an optimal emotional "match." (Where one, for example, was reserved, the other may have been demonstrative; where one was adventurous, the other may have been timid.) And sometimes it is simply that they have never come to terms with the fact that their mothers were not the superhuman, omnipotent beings they wanted them to be.

In any case, during pregnancy, women who have the most complaints about their mothers are the ones who most often obsess on the notion that they will turn into their mothers, or rather *into the worst parts of their mothers*, when their new babies arrive. Ask them what it is they fear most and the responses run quite a gamut: Being "hysterical," being "tyrannical," being "weak," being "rigid," being "overwhelmed," being "too emotional," being "cold."

Images of their mothers at their most vexatious visit these pregnant women's psyches as their babies bounce around inside their bellies. While an expectant mother lies awake, the images can upset her so greatly that she may find herself sobbing into her pillow or clutching the bed sheets in terror of re-creating her own mother's troublesome traits and becoming the latest in a long line of "neurotic" mothers. When she is asleep, the same images can become the stuff of nightmares:

> "I dreamed that when I had the baby I was back living with my parents," recalled 24-year-old Ellyn. "The baby was crying and my mother pulled me away when I tried to comfort the child. She kept saying, 'Just leave her alone, and she'll stop.' Then *I* started crying uncontrollably, and my mother turned and ran away from me."

When asked what she thought this dream signified, Ellyn replied:

> "My mother always told me she couldn't cope with the sound of my crying when I was an infant. She said sometimes she left me in my crib, closed the door, and turned on the radio to drown me out. I hated those stories. I wish she would have held that little girl that was me. But to tell the truth, the sound of kids' crying upsets me too. I worried, would I have to do what she did?"

Forty-year-old Sarah recalled:

"I dreamed my mother came over to visit my new baby, and when I was out of the room she took the baby and hid him behind his crib. I came back and found him. I was horrified. I asked her why she had done this, and she said it was because she didn't want the neighbors to see that his ears were big and that he was not as 'pretty' as his older brother."

When asked what this dream called up for her, Sarah responded:

"I think I dreamed this because I'd always had the feeling from my mother that she didn't love me as much as my older sister. I know I was afraid that I would play favorites now that I was having a second child."

But then, Sarah confessed another fear, one that a fair number of expectant mothers owned up to:

"On the other hand, I have to admit that part of me thinks I will do whatever I have to do to make sure my kids are treated very differently than I was treated. But instead of feeling virtuous and proud of myself for that, I sometimes am a bit resentful. I feel cheated. I wish I had been given what I am about to give."

Many mothers-to-be who carry grievances about their childhoods face just such an emotional conundrum. They are partly afraid of becoming prisoners of family history, repeating what went before. But they are also aware that if they manage to do otherwise, they might have to face envying their children for receiving something which they themselves were denied. If this seems a paradox, mothers-to-be might as well get used to it. For it is one of many paradoxical situations that motherhood presents to women who are in touch with their own emotions and honest enough to acknowledge them. Life as a mother will always be psychologically demanding—but it will never be dull.

Of course, an expectant mother can try her best not to think about quickening and all its ramifications. She may resist processing the fact that her imaginary baby is coming closer and closer to its "coming out" party. Or she can think of that child only in terms of traits she deems ideal. (Let's hear it for that adorable, ever-cooing miracle baby who sleeps all night and composes piano sonatas by day.) Similarly, she can take the Pollyanna Pregnant path and allow herself to consciously experience only pie-in-the-sky fantasies of motherhood and all its virtues and charms. (Let's hear it for that perennially patient, constantly cuddling miracle mother who bakes cookies all night while her baby sleeps and accompanies his or her piano sonatas on the violin before breakfast.)

But if she does much of this, she may be unpleasantly surprised by her complex reactions to the reality of the baby after birth. For no baby is "ideal" just as no mother is "ideal," and hence no relationship between them can be so. (As many a woman has noted in hindsight, "I was the perfect mother, until I became one.") Better to let the quickening herald, as it would seem it is naturally meant to, a new phase of the pregnancy: a phase in which a woman develops an ever-increasing awareness of her womb-mate and begins to grapple more deeply than before with her own issues about the tasks of mothering that lie before her.

As so many expectant mothers make clear, sheer joy is a part of what the quickening brings. Beginning each day with happy anticipation of when the baby will kick up its heels is generally one of the most pleasurable aspects of pregnancy's middle trimester. But self-doubt is also part of the process, and a healthy part at that, providing one uses it as a tool for self-awareness rather than a weapon aimed directly at one's own head.

Try not to burden yourself with unrealistic expectations or compulsions when it comes to evaluating your parenting skills. Yes, you may be, at times, high-strung or short-tempered or what have you. And you may at times even act—gasp!—like your mother on one of her less than magnificent days. But your baby does not require that you have a personality transplant, or that you do all good things all of the time. Your child only requires, as the pediatrician and psychoanalyst D. W. Winnicott has noted, that you be a "good enough" parent, that you offer your baby a variety of experiences, with an aim not to eliminate frustration (since frustration is an inevitable part of life for babies and adults alike), but to incorporate it in an emotional environment that is *overall* affectionate and accepting.

Your imaginary baby, so soon to leave your womb, will not—no matter what you may envision—emerge wearing a tiny judicial robe and carrying a gavel, ready to pronounce sentence upon you. He or she will emerge ready to hold on to you and give you every chance, and then some, to love him or her in all his or her "realness." As he or she will love you in all of yours.

❖ AN EXPECTANT MOTHER'S PRIVILEGES
AND PREROGATIVES

Have fun making contact. Feeling your baby move may make you feel like beginning to sing to him, make small talk with him, or even read to him. It may make you feel like playing music for her, or burning a fragrant candle for her, or stroking and caressing her through your own skin. While it's fascinating to speculate about how much of this stimulation will be *re*ceived or *per*ceived by your child, don't worry so much about that. Instead, if it feels good do it. Gently saying "hi" to your baby in your own special way is, at the very least, good therapy for *you*.

On the other hand, only make as much contact as feels right for you. Don't let others pressure you into trying to "program" your baby to be born loving Mozart or speaking French. And don't let them make you feel guilty if you're too sleepy to croon a lullaby to your in vivo baby each and every night. It doesn't mean you've failed the Parent Test.

Note your "hunches" and your dreams in your journal. Midpregnancy, the time of quickening, is, if you'll pardon the pun, a very fertile time. It will be very interesting to see what comes up for you in terms of ideas you have about your baby—his or her gender, his appearance, her personality traits, and so on. It will also be very enlightening to see what comes up for you in terms of thoughts or anxieties you have concerning your own mothering capabilities. (You might try asking yourself: What aspects of motherhood do you think will challenge you the most? What do you think your strong suits are in terms of parenting? In what ways would you like most to influence your child?) Writing about all this will help you to clarify your expectations of motherhood and help you begin to process the "reality" of your baby.

When you have "premonitions" about your baby, or dreams about him or her or about your role as a parent, try noting these too down in your journal. This should help you get a handle on the many mixed emotions that may be stirred up by all this psychic activity.

If you find you are having trouble writing (maybe you've never thought of yourself as much of a writer) don't feel you have to be confined to linear sentences and paragraphs. Making lists is a perfectly fine alternative way of compiling thoughts or images. So is drawing a circle around a central idea or feeling you'd like to express and then at the ends of arrows drawn radiating outward from the circle (as you might draw the rays of the sun) writing in any associations you have to that central concept.

Don't worry that expressing your feelings might harm the baby. Remember back to when you first discovered you were pregnant. Like a lot of women, you probably wondered then if any doubts or fears you had at that time might do damage to the tiny embryo inside you. It wasn't so then and it isn't so now.

Your baby has some sensory perception. How much it's not certain. But even if, for argument's sake, we say that your baby may be able to "feel" your state of mind, do you think it will benefit him or her to have you continually struggling to censor your naturally occurring thoughts?

It is true some studies indicate that women under extreme and constant stress can, through increased production of adrenaline and noradrenaline, induce a stressful state in their babies (leading to lower birth weights, prematurity, or hyperactivity).[6] But repressing your feelings is far more likely to induce a physiologically stressful state than processing them and letting them meet the light of day. What you express in words is less likely to be expressed by bodily agitation.

Share your fears—and have some laughs—with other expectant mothers. Fears about having shortcomings as a mother are so widespread during pregnancy that a down-and-dirty discussion with your network of cohorts will make you feel better. At the very least, you will know you are not alone. At best, you may find your universal theme not only a source of solace but an occasional source of mirth. Exactly what sort of madwoman do you picture yourself becoming once you're in the grips of motherhood? Will you become the terror of your local supermarket? The pariah of the PTA? Chances are your compatriots will have even more garish and—when viewed in a certain convivial spirit—more hilarious visions than yours. You'll find there is nothing like the salve of humor to take the sting out of anxiety.

Vow only to be a good enough mother. No matter how altruistic you'd like to be, the reality is that you are a mere mortal. Mortals make mistakes and often are a cause of frustration to other mortals—of which your child will be one. Do not buy into the fallacy that only those with the saintly temperament of a Divine Mother can make adequate parents here in the earthly realm. Aim only to be a good enough mother of the lowercase *m* variety.

Give your own mother a break. When you were a small child in a big world, your mother seemed very large indeed. It was only natural from your perspective to exaggerate her good qualities, as well as the ones which you found disappointing. Now, on the threshold of having a child and facing all the huge unknowns that child will introduce, it is also easy, and perfectly normal, to sometimes feel very "small." So once again your mother's frustrating qualities can take on a kind of immensity.

Try to restore some perspective to the situation. Remember, if you can, the positive aspects of the way your mother mothered. (There must have been some, or you wouldn't be here, let alone be functioning the way you do.)

To brand your mother as nothing but a villain will not prove helpful to you at any time, but especially not now. It will prevent you from seeking any nurturing from her at a time when you yourself could doubtless use some mothering. (If you give her a chance, she may rise to the occasion in ways that surprise you.) It also devalues her, which in turn devalues you—because whatever else you are, you are also a part of her, as the baby somersaulting inside you now is part of you. To deny your mother's fundamental good intentions (regardless of your relationship's sore points) is to devalue all mothers, all women, who struggle—as you will have to—with the very real and numerous emotional challenges of caring for and raising a child and, ultimately, letting that child go his or her own way.

One more thing: Thinking, dreaming, and fantasizing about your baby, and ruminating about what it means to be a mother is all a very necessary part of the pregnancy process. But it tends to be extremely preoccupying, sometimes too much so. An expectant mother needs to remember that the bond between her and her baby also extends to include another. In the next chapter we'll see what fathers-to-be are thinking and feeling at this point, and how pregnancy can affect the dynamics of couples.

6 The Pregnant Husband

All three of us are tied in this heart, this belly.

—GLADYS HINDMARCH
A Birth Account

When my husband and I first started telling people we were expecting a baby, we would say proudly, "We're pregnant." Obviously, I knew there were parts of the process that would fall exclusively into my domain, just as there were parts that would fall into his. (I wasn't going to be doing much lifting and hauling, for example, when we moved into the new house we were buying in honor of the baby's arrival.) Still, in our minds at this early stage this was, in nearly every sense, a joint endeavor. And so we continued to say to friends and family and colleagues and to one another, "We're pregnant."

Together, as the months went on, we tackled many of the logistical and emotional challenges with which our pregnancy presented us. We planned, we packed, we purchased. We wondered. We worried. We tossed and turned. Every night, my partner rubbed my inflating tummy with massage ointment. Every month, he attended my prenatal exam, listened to his child's boisterous heartbeat, and shot the breeze with my midwife. He made sure I ate leafy greens. He gave up *caffeine with me. Most important of all, he couldn't have been more enthusiastic about the prospect of parenthood, and he promised sincerely that he would participate fully in the rearing of our little one from the moment he poked his tiny head into the world.*

By the sixth month of pregnancy, our unborn child had already brought us closer in countless ways. It was such an awesome concept creating a new being—half him, half me—that words often failed. Even then, being mutually dumbstruck turned out to be a most binding emotional affixative.

Undeniably, though, there were also other kinds of feelings. And as the months passed they took hold in me more and more strongly.

Sometimes, when my husband was so understanding about whatever particular pregnancy-related mania was plaguing me at the moment, I felt a mild urge to scream, "Don't patronize me!"

Sometimes, when he was ever so slightly late coming home from work I had visions of great harm befalling him. I would pace the floor envisioning his fatal brush with a tractor trailer. Part of me was genuinely petrified to face my fate as a widowed mother; part of me was agitated at my own paranoia, not to mention my sense of helplessness and overdependence.

Sometimes I felt frustrated with this spousal paragon simply because no matter how empathic and caring and concerned my husband was, he wasn't the one carrying the baby inside him, was he?

Okay, there you have it. He wasn't the one whose clothes didn't fit anymore and whose fingers were swelling. He wasn't the one forbidden to have a cognac after dinner (not that he did, but he could have, you see). He wasn't the one befuddled to the variety of breast pumps on the market. And, hey, he wasn't the one who was going to have to push a great, big bouncing baby through a teeny-weeny birth canal. He was getting off easy.

As much as I love my husband and wanted to share everything with him, in some senses I knew there were places I was

*about to go where he could not follow. Sometimes it seemed
so unfair. Sometimes it made me lonely. Funny thing was, he
said—and I believed him—that if Mother Nature had been
more equality-minded he would have been happy to be the
one to carry the child, the one to give birth, the one to nurse.*

*I think the fact that he wasn't able to be pregnant in the
literal sense made him lonely sometimes too. . . .*

A Pregnant Husband's Tasks

If there were such a thing as an ideal expectant father—according
to most expectant mothers, that is—he would have a list of laud-
able traits that matched or exceeded those of the Boy Scout credo.
He would be trustworthy, loyal, helpful, friendly, courteous, kind,
cheerful, and brave. Beyond that he would be patient, indulgent,
reassuring, curious, concerned, and—above all—empathic and
involved.

Like a Scout, he would be devoted to doing "good turns" on
a regular basis. Among those he would have begun doing in the
first and second trimester are these:

❖ He would have responded to his wife's reaction to pregnancy so that she felt supported and understood. (As we
saw earlier, women like to feel their husbands' emotions
resonating with their own as they process the momentous
news. They don't want to be "talked out" of having their
particular feelings, whatever they may be.)

❖ He would have been clear that he was dealing with a wife
in the throes of emotional and hormonal upheaval and
treated her not like she was crazy, but like she was pregnant. (Among the Basongye of Zaire, men say they know
a woman is pregnant when she is always angry. And in
Busama, New Guinea, they believe it is critical to let a
pregnant wife win every argument.[1] Such bits of wisdom
are obviously a bit extreme, but most wives agree a certain
amount of leeway for the vacillations of the pregnant temperament couldn't hurt.)

❖ He would have learned a fair amount about the process of pregnancy and birth so that he could participate in making informed choices. (Because education should not begin and end with the expectant mother.)

❖ He would have tried to accompany his partner to at least some of her medical exams and to get to know her practitioner. (Because three heads are often better than two, and a husband may well think of questions and considerations that might not have occurred to his wife.)

❖ He would have expressed sincerely and frequently that his wife's changing body was beautiful to him. (Demi Moore said that was *her* secret.)

❖ He would have supported his wife's efforts to lead a healthy life-style, and what's more he would have joined her in it. (In other words, he'd understand it is unseemly to taunt or tempt a pregnant woman with a heaping platter of sour creamed burritos while she is grazing at the salad bar.)

❖ He would have begun eagerly anticipating his role as a new father. (He'd accept that today this role goes beyond making funny faces and bouncing the baby on his knee and instead includes everything from changing diapers to drying tears.)

❖ He would have adjusted without complaint to his wife's changing sexual desires and done all he could to accommodate her in that area. (As we'll see, this means different things to different couples, as some women's sexual desire increases during pregnancy, while others' decreases.)

As the pregnancy progresses into its final trimester, the tasks of the expectant father compound. Ideally, he would continue to refine his prior duties, while mastering these additional ones:

❖ He will be an enthusiastic attender of prepared childbirth classes. (Valiantly learning about such things as contractions effacement, dilatation, and crowning—all without flinching.)

❖ He will prepare himself to be the perfect labor coach, laying in his sipper cup, stopwatch, and massage manual, rehearsing his pep talks, and polishing his delivery room etiquette. (No fainting or shrieking for him.)

❖ He will do as much as he can to help his wife remain as physically comfortable as possible as the time of child-birth approaches. (This can include everything from rubbing her sciatica to helping her tie her shoes or shave her legs when she can no longer bend over.)

❖ He will also help her remain as emotionally comfortable as possible, being more tolerant than ever of her concerns about her body, her moods, her fears of managing—or indeed of surviving—labor and delivery, and her anxieties about mothering. (In short the father-to-be will "mother" his wife in the best way he knows how.)

Remember this lengthy list of duties is expected to be performed—indeed perfectly executed—by the *ideal* pregnant husband. But what about real flesh-and-blood thinking-and-feeling pregnant husbands? Are they up to these various and sundry jobs? Incredible as it may seem, many do amazingly well in their roles as nurturers to their wives, fathers-in-training, prepared childbirth students, and the like. Many contemporary women gave their pregnant husbands high marks for their efforts on all or most fronts. They often remarked as well that, based on discussions with their own mothers, they believed their husbands were involved in the pregnancy process to a far greater extent than their fathers had ever been.

Yet many also had a sense that certain things remained unspoken. They perceived their husbands as "taking a backseat" in decision-making, or "biting their tongues" when they felt afraid or frustrated. Even if asked if something was troubling them, they might well deny it or defuse the question by making some sort of self-deprecating joke. It was as if, some of the time, their husbands were suppressing some of their own feelings on behalf of what was generally perceived as the greater good, i.e., the equanimity of the expectant mother.

I wondered what toll such suppression may be taking on fathers-to-be, and what they would say if they felt free to say everything. As it turned out, many of them, though sincerely pleased to be as helpful as possible to their pregnant wives, felt frustrated too. They found the many expectations that their spouses, and society in general, had of them difficult to contend with. And they believed themselves to be the recipients of some perplexing and nerve-racking mixed messages.

A Pregnant Husband's Trials

Consider the basic, underlying mixed message that is given to the contemporary pregnant husband. According to today's cultural ethic, fatherhood is chic, paternal presence at birthing classes and birth itself is politically correct, and "real men" think it's cool to cut the umbilical cord. In short, immersement in every aspect of the pregnancy and childbirth process is the "in" thing. Pregnant wives reinforce the premise in many ways. They remind their men that they're in this together, as in many senses they truly are. But not in every sense, *not exactly.*

This *not exactly* clause makes for a touchy predicament as far as men are concerned. The same society which encourages them to be full participants in the miracle denies them some of the fringe benefits available to their *literally* pregnant wives. Most of the accoutrements and rituals of pregnancy—the maternity wardrobe, the baby shower, the prenatal exams, the solicitous phone calls from friends and relations, and the knowing smiles—revolve around the wife. And pregnant husbands, of course, do not "show," hence strangers have no means of identifying them in order to grant them small pregnancy "perks."

But even among those who know an expectant father's situation, few cut him much slack. They don't recognize that pregnant husbands often have as many personal preoccupations clamoring for space in their minds as do their wives, and that their sleep quotient tends to diminish in direct proportion to that of their fitfully tossing, up-five-times-to-go-to-the-bathroom mates.

Even pregnant wives themselves sometimes find it difficult to give guys a break when the men are, say, moody or anxious or exhausted or less than wholly rational. Ironically, some of the same women who insist on their husband's full empathic involvement often draw a line should their spouses' symptoms start to mimic their own too closely. In a pinch, the wife will hasten to remind him that only one of them is the actual child-bearer here. While this may be accurate, expectant fathers can find it an irritating brand of oneupmanship (or, more correctly, oneupwomanship).

So the typical 1990s pregnant husband, delighted as he may be to find himself in the evolved, enlightened role of caretaker of mother and child, sometimes finds himself wondering who is supposed to take care of him. Clearly, this is a time when many of his needs are, perhaps necessarily, put on the back burner. And even though that may genuinely be okay with him, the dearth of compensatory fanfare and kudos that accompanies his sacrifice is not lost on him.

In other cultures throughout history pregnant fathers have had rituals of their own, which were known as "couvade" (from the French verb *couver,* which means to brood or hatch). Sometimes couvade entailed observing various prohibitions, such as abstaining from certain foods or stopping work and going into seclusion as the time of the baby's delivery neared. Often it entailed pseudo-labor type behavior on the father's part, meaning that even as his wife was delivering their child, the husband would writhe, pant, and moan as if he too were birthing a baby.

Anthropologists have long speculated about the reasons for couvade's existence. It is believed by some that primitive cultures used it to divert the attention of evil spirits away from the pregnant woman herself, so that she would remain safe. It is believed by others that couvade was begun when the link between sex and pregnancy was poorly understood, as a means of establishing a link between a husband and his wife's child.[2] In addition, however, couvade would seem surely to have served an important psychological need for the father-to-be. Through his appointed rituals he too gained attention and respect. He too was granted a privileged and special position in his family and in his community.

We have no ritual couvade in which expectant fathers routinely participate. Instead we have couvade "syndrome," the psychological term which describes fathers-to-be who (some-what preposterously, we seem to think) exhibit weight gain, bloating, nausea, or lack of appetite. On a more humorous note, we also have a trendy gag known as the "Empathy Belly," which pregnant men are laughingly told they can "try on for size" if they want to know what it's really like to carry a child to term. (The device weighs 35 pounds, and as Jessica Mitford describes, it "is guaranteed to cause backache, shortness of breath, and fatigue, and comes with a special pouch on the wearer's bladder, creating an uncomfortable desire to urinate at inappropriate moments.")[3]

What a bind the pregnant husband is in. On a physical level, he is supposed to identify with his wife, but if he does so too much, he is derided. Alas, the same holds true for his psychological identification.

As a result of their being *not exactly* pregnant, many men feel that any discussion of the reservations and fears which are wholly natural at this juncture in their lives would be welcome only up to a point. They are often reluctant to speak—because they don't feel they have permission to say anything that is less than one hundred percent sensitive, supportive, and maritally correct.

However, when prompted (and assured that names would be changed to protect the innocent) these are the sort of sentiments they revealed:

"I want to be a good father to my kids, a dad who is really actively involved, who they will really know cares and who is *around*," said 37-year-old Edward. "But I'm afraid I will fail at this, because I had no role model for being this kind of father. My own dad was distant emotionally. It was so hard to get his attention. And he was often distant physically, because his job required a lot of travel. My job requires some travel too, though not as much, but still I'm aware that my boss isn't going to care that I've got a baby at home if a business trip is required. As far as my work world is concerned, a new dad hands out cigars and gets on with his business. If I started talking about feeling conflicted I'm afraid it might be pro-fessional suicide."

"I worry that once the baby comes my wife won't have time for me anymore," said 33-year-old Luke. "We're both so busy now, but she always seems to find time to plan a little romance. I'm a realist. I know a baby will disrupt all our routines and demand so much of us both, but especially of her in the beginning. I'm afraid that the baby will take my place in her heart, that she won't have room enough or time enough for two of us. But what a jerk I might sound like if I told her!"

"For me the big fear is that something will happen to my wife during pregnancy or childbirth, that some harm will come to her," confided 29-year-old Jim. "I know that's highly unlikely, but it doesn't prevent me from dwelling on morbid thoughts sometimes. On days when she's not feeling so great, it's especially hard. I really want to help her, but how much can I actually do? Of course I would never say any of this to her. I feel it's my place to act optimistic and assured all the time."

"My concern is about being this supposedly great labor coach," confessed 44-year-old Benjamin. "Everyone, most of all my wife, just seems to assume that I will be equipped, after a handful of 'prepared childbirth' classes and a couple of videotapes, to instruct her while *she's* having our baby. I'm supposed to help her relax, right? But what if I'm a nervous wreck myself? What if I panic? I have recurrent nightmares about standing in the delivery room unable to speak, paralyzed, while doctors and nurses yell at me to do something useful or get out. To me, it is the ultimate performance anxiety. I guess, to be honest, I resent the fact that no one ever really asked me if I thought I would be good at this. But how can I say this when, after all, it is my wife who has the really hard job ahead?"

Certainly expectant fathers have feelings other than doubts or fears. Like their wives, they often have all kinds of upbeat, pleasurable thoughts about what it will be like to add a new member to their family. But, also like their wives, they can feel conflicted some of the time. They too find that childhood memories emerge as a potent force in their consciousness during pregnancy, perhaps for the first time in a long time. And they find their dreams are chock-full of imagery concerning pregnancy, birth, and impending parenthood. Yet a reluctance to discuss any of these natural emotional phenomena is a powerful shared theme among fathers-to-be.

Many men feel it is simply *never* alright to let anyone know what kinds of things are really troubling them as a pregnancy proceeds. Some feel it is only permissible to worry publicly about what society tends to deem appropriate masculine provinces, for instance the financial ramifications of familyhood and the potential loss of freedom—to pursue hobbies, sports, and so forth—that tending a baby will entail. (In actuality, these particular concerns may be of equal weight to both genders, but stereotypical perceptions often prevail as to who ought to officially worry about what.)

On most other matters, though, silence reigns. For pregnant fathers believe they have an image to keep up, at home, at work, at doctor's visits, and even—perhaps especially—in those prepared childbirth classes where they are expected, in the course of a few months or weeks, to transform themselves from neophytes into bona fide experts in a matter that is as complex and challenging emotionally as it is physically. Couple this dynamic of bravado with a wife who doesn't quite swallow the idea that her husband is in as much of an altered state as she, and it becomes understandable why communication problems sometimes develop between a father-to-be and a mother-to-be.

The Pregnant Couple, the Changing Bond

The best way for couples to navigate through the pregnancy months is for both parties to regularly remind themselves that they are both, in their own separate but equal ways, pregnant. They are equal in the sense that to be pregnant means full, fertile, prolific, teeming with meaning and significance. They are separate in the sense that every pregnancy has both yin and yang (that is, female and male) aspects. Both are necessary, both are valuable. But neither one is precisely like the other.

Certainly a loving, cooperative husband ought to be understanding, compassionate, and supportive of his wife, while doing his best to empathize with her female perspective on the pregnancy. But your job description, as it relates to your husband, ought to be much the same. You need to draw your husband out, hear him out, and try to empathize with his masculine perspective on your joint endeavor. At times when neither of you, no matter how hard you try, truly comprehends the other's point of view (as is wont to happen in any marriage from time to time, and is almost inevitable when a couple is in the midst of all the changes involved in the course of a pregnancy) that still need not preclude you from respecting the fact that a valid point of view other than your own does exist.

Each milestone of pregnancy—the discovery of conception, the public acknowledgment, the decision-making process concerning prenatal care, the baby's "showing," the first signs of quickening, the nesting impulses, the childbirth classes, the labor and birth itself—affects each partner in profound ways. But they may not and need not be the same ways.

To a pregnant woman, for example, beginning to "show" may lead to feelings of self-doubt about her attractiveness. To her husband, it may lead to feelings of pride about his virility, his "job well done." To an expectant mother, imagining a delivery at which the father's role is that of head coach may feel comforting. To an expectant father, it may feel like an unnerving prospect.

Neither person is "crazy" or "wrong" for having the feelings they have. But what would be wrong would be to act on those feelings in a way that shuts the other party out. Better to use the powerful emotions of pregnancy constructively whenever possible.

A husband who scoffs that his wife's insecurity about her pregnant body is vain and frivolous will do her and their relationship little good. Whereas one who reassures her by telling her how lovely she is to him, and how proud she makes him by carrying his child, will immeasurably improve her frame of mind and brighten the household atmosphere. Likewise, a wife who complains that her husband's hesitancy to take on a coaching task brands him as unsympathetic or cowardly will do less to pave the way for an emotionally satisfying labor experience than one who takes the time to notice whether her spouse is looking rather pale and panicky during those up close and personal delivery room videos and asks him to tell her in what way *he'd* be most comfortable participating in the experience.

It may sound academic to suggest that expectant mothers and fathers exercise thoughtfulness and diplomacy in their interactions with one another. Obviously such practices benefit any relationship at any time. And it's quite likely a husband and wife have mastered such niceties to some extent to have gotten to the point where they are having a family together. But the advent of a new baby creates anomalies in the natural flow of things. It is a totally new and untried cog in the well-oiled machine that is an existent marriage. And it mandates that certain lessons be relearned and adapted to fit present circumstances.

Once the baby actually arrives, its impact on the marriage will be enormous. It is actually fortunate then that the pregnancy months offer bountiful opportunities to rehearse dealing with one's spouse not only as a partner but as a fellow parent, i.e., as someone consumed with forging a special bond with a brand-new, totally unknown, extremely high-maintenance being.

As month after month of pregnancy marches by, shared practical concerns will demand more and more of a couple's attention. Will there be, for example, enough living space and enough money to go around? Shared emotional concerns will also be major focal points. For example, will there be enough love to go around? Though expectant mothers and fathers may respond to such critical concerns in their own particular fashions (perhaps one optimistically, one more pessimistically; or one with jokes and one with tears), it is important to remember that each is trying to cope with stress in the best way he or she knows how.

With the right attitude, you will find there will be many times when it will help to laugh and cry together, and to recognize that disparate responses are often two sides of one coin. Ask couples who have been through it and they will tell you that those times of mutual openness and acceptance (such as saying what each of you *really* thinks after seeing one of those infamous childbirth videotapes or admitting to each other just how baffled you are about what you'll actually do with this baby of yours once you get it home) will be the source of some of your fondest pregnancy memories.

A Word About Sex

For couples who do manage to solicit and accept each other's feelings, the pregnancy months can be a time of deepening intimacy. But there is one form of intimacy that many fear relinquishing as the pregnancy advances—and that, of course, is the sexual aspect of marriage.

Though most people today like to think of themselves as fairly sophisticated when it comes to matters of sex, sexuality during pregnancy is one area where an extraordinary number of myths and misconceptions abound. It is easy to see why. Many expectant couples rely on snippets of information they picked up here and there. Then they feel that something is amiss if their own reality does not conform to what they've heard.

> "My best friend told me that pregnancy was a time when a woman felt maternal, but not sexual," said Marlene, pregnant with her first child at age 27. "She said it was a chemical thing. You can imagine my surprise when I felt more interested in sex than ever. I felt so aroused, but you know I was shy about telling my husband. I honestly thought there must be something wrong with me, that this was some sort of deviant behavior or something."

> "Before we started having kids, I heard that pregnant women were very sexually oriented, something or other about their hormones going wild," said 34-year-old Jeffrey. "But my wife, who's now

pregnant with our third child, has never qualified as living proof of this assertion.

"I keep waiting for her to hear the same rumors as me. But no matter how many times she gets pregnant, she doesn't want to do anything in bed except sleep."

"We heard that it was completely safe to have sex during pregnancy, and that it was a good idea to do so because it was relaxing and because it would help prepare the uterus and pelvic muscles for birth," said Regina and Jim, who were expecting their first child while they both were on the verge of turning 40. "But as the birth gets closer we both feel nervous about sex possibly harming the baby or bringing on premature labor, which we've also heard was possible. Maybe we're being overly cautious. But now [at nearly the seventh month] we just kiss and hug a lot. Which is okay by us . . . but, I don't know, do you think it's because we're old fogies?"

Interestingly, none of these people is, technically speaking, suffering from *mis*information. And none of their behaviors or feelings are unusual, let alone aberrant. They simply don't realize how many physical, emotional, and aesthetic variants there are when it comes to pregnancy and sexuality.

It is true that during pregnancy levels of the female sex hormone estriol (a type of estrogen) increase. It is also true that female genitals increase in size and that there is an increase in vaginal secretions, both of which phenomena are also indicative of physiological feminine sexual arousal.[4] Based on these facts, it's easy to see why some conclude physical factors will predispose pregnant women to have a heightened interest in sex.

But consider also that the levels of free-ranging testosterone in a woman's body decrease during pregnancy. (According to some sexologists, this hormone contributes a great deal to the sex drive in women.)[5] Consider also that toward the end of pregnancy the vagina can become so swollen that orgasmic contractions become very difficult to sense. And the movement of the baby itself may be distracting. And breasts may be painfully tender. Based on these facts, one could easily construct a strictly physical rationale as to why pregnant women might experience a decrease in sexual interest.

Now, of course, it is imperative to take into account emotional factors which superimpose themselves on physiological ones. For example, a desire to connect with one's partner during this special time, or simply to relax and take one's mind off things, may stoke the sex drive. So might the very notion that previous sex has resulted in living proof of a couple's potency.

> "Our sex life during pregnancy was absolutely wonderful," said 38-year-old Grant. "I think both of us were turned on by the idea that, hey, we must be good at this. We've got a baby to show for it! Every time I looked at my wife I felt extremely virile and masculine. And every time she looked in the mirror, she was reminded of her femininity. We were really 'charged.'"

On the other hand, anxiety about hurting the baby or about the upcoming birth itself or about the burdens of motherhood may detract from the sex drive (anxiety being to sex what a heat wave is to a snow sculpture). And when a woman feels unattractive because of her changing body shape and weight gain this too, not surprisingly, can put a damper on romance.

> "With each pound I gained I felt more reluctant to show myself to my husband," confessed 33-year-old Tess. "I became more and more hesitant to become intimate. I wish I could say it had been otherwise, but I had difficulty breaking the connection in my mind between sexiness and slenderness."

To all this add the aesthetic inclinations of both partners. As the pregnancy progresses, it's often necessary to be somewhat inventive when it comes to such matters as sexual positioning. It may also be necessary to change the time of day when sex is on the agenda, because evening may bring fatigue, whereas morning may bring nausea. Some couples find such variations a turn-on, while some find them just the opposite.

All in all, it is not startling to see why some studies note a marked increase in sexual activity among couples expecting a baby, while others record exactly the opposite tendency. There is no "norm." It all depends on which couples one asks. And it may even depend on *when* one asks them, for it is not unusual for a couple's sexual activity to change significantly as a pregnancy proceeds toward its conclusion and as different sorts of emotions wax and wane.

Theories and studies aside, what is most important for mother- and father-to-be to know is that, after consulting your doctor or midwife (who will most likely advise that it is fine to have sex during pregnancy, but in some "second line" cases caution against intercourse for part or all of the pregnancy), it is up to you, in patient, loving communication with one another, to create a sexual scenario that is comfortable for you both, without regard to what anyone else in your situation has (allegedly) done or not done.

As with all joint decisions, discussions of sexuality need to take into account the points of view and feelings of both people involved. It is easy to see where one partner's reluctance to have sex—perhaps out of fear or embarrassment or out of what he or she believes is consideration for a spouse—can be misinterpreted as a personal rejection if it is not explained. A little dialogue will go a long way toward avoiding such misunderstandings. And whatever you decide about sex—or anything else—a lot of plain old snuggling will go a long way toward making everyone feel loved.

❖ AN EXPECTANT MOTHER'S PRIVILEGES AND PREROGATIVES

Tell him what you need, ask him what he needs. Certainly you have an obligation to yourself and to the child you are carrying to be clear during your pregnancy about what it is you need from your spouse in order to be comfortable emotionally during this time of great change and anticipation. But you also have an obligation to your husband and to your marriage. In the past, it probably never would have seemed fair to you if you got to call all the shots in your relationship. Well, it still isn't fair. If you want your relationship to thrive (and you can give your child no better gift) you've simply got to solicit input from your partner as to how he would like to participate along with you in the pregnancy, birth, and parenting experience.

Give a pregnant guy a break. Couvade is alive and well. Though in our day and age we are not much concerned with the warding off of evil spirits, and though husbands are not wont to writhe and moan while their wives go through labor, numerous fathers-to-be still seem to develop physical and emotional symptoms very similar to those of their pregnant wives. If your husband does this, it is best not to belittle or mock his symptoms (be they exhaustion, weight gain, mood swings, or a more serious case of infirmity). In part, his manifestations represent his overwhelming identification with you. But in part, they likely also represent his legitimate need for attention and mothering.

Giving him just that to the extent you can manage it would be a good idea. You may as well practice mothering now, as you'll be doing lots of it later. What's more, making a bit of a fuss over your spouse on occasion can help you get your mind off whatever concerns may be nagging at you. And if you've been feeling like the helpless or clinging one in the relationship, this should make you feel less so.

Reassure him a lot. You know the way you sometimes fear that things will change in your marriage once a new baby arrives, and that your husband will have less time and affection to give to you? Your husband probably feels exactly the same way, even if he doesn't verbalize it. Reminding him often how much you care about him will not only make him feel good, but will likely elicit similar reassurances from him. And wouldn't that be nice? Consider your efforts a form of enlightened self-interest.

Suggest rituals for him. Remember, your husband doesn't get much public affirmation for being pregnant. He doesn't get to be cooed over at the maternity store, and no one tells him he's "radiant." Perhaps you can be of help in rectifying this situation to some degree. You might want to consider organizing a "Daddy shower" for him (or at least making your own shower a coed affair). You might want to suggest that he get together with other men whose wives are pregnant or who are new dads, in a kind of ad hoc support group.

You can also think of ways in which your partner can turn his nervous energy into creative energy, suggesting that he might want to be in charge of designing a personalized birth announcement or constructing a piece of furniture for the nursery. (And whatever emerges from his efforts, be certain to *adore* it.)

Make sure your caregivers care for your husband too. Unfortunately many fathers-to-be voiced the opinion that their wives' prenatal practitioners, while welcoming their participation in theory, did not welcome it as much in deed. If you and your husband want to share in as much of the pregnancy and childbirth experience as possible, choose a doctor or midwife who is as enthusiastic about the plan as you are, and who gives it more than lip service. You will know, early on, from the nature of the interactions between your practitioner and your spouse whether or not your partner is made to feel welcome. Does your husband have to stand during appointments because no chair is provided for him? Is he treated cooly or condescendingly? Is he ignored while all comments and questions are addressed to you? If so, discuss with your caregiver how you would like your husband to be acknowledged. If he or she won't oblige you, find a practitioner who will.

Ask how your spouse sees his role at the birth. Nowadays many couples simply assume that the employment of a husband as a labor coach is the thing to do. There is no question that many couples have found husband-coached childbirth a deeply rewarding experience for all parties involved, but don't *assume* that is what will suit you both best without doing some thinking and talking about it first. *Ask your husband:* Does he feel comfortable not only guiding you through the birth process, but acting as your advocate and being responsible for conveying your wishes to the hospital staff? Will he feel comfortable doing all this while he himself is feeling an immense, intense emotional involvement in what is going on?

If, after educating yourselves about what a labor coach does, you and your partner decide he's the coach you both want, go for it. But if you or he are not totally sold on the idea, consider other options. Engaging a trained professional labor coach or childbirth assistant to support you and your husband through the birth is one option you ought to seriously consider. (See this book's Resource List for help in finding one.) If you do this, it can free up your husband to minister to you emotionally, without having to feel the added stresses of doing all those other jobs.

Whatever you decide, allowing your partner to be present at the birth in a way that feels appropriate and comfortable for him will make for a more agreeable experience all around.

Expand your definition of sexuality and intimacy. As pregnancy progresses, you may find that, for any number of reasons, your sex life undergoes various changes. Perhaps you are not having intercourse as much as before, perhaps not at all. But this time should not be looked on as a time of decrease, but as an opportunity for increase. You may well find that other paths to physical gratification (meaning anything from hugging, stroking, and massaging to methods of sexual fulfillment which don't involve intercourse) can be exceptionally rewarding. And you will likely also find that, on an emotional level, you and your partner can use the pregnancy period to learn more about each other than ever before.

This is a time to treat each other gently and respectfully, but also to take some risks, to expose your vulnerabilities, to explore your roles in the relationship. It is an excellent chance to widen the lens through which you perceive each other and your life together. It is also a time to bask in the comfort of sharing an awesome experience with someone who knows you so very well. Especially since, as we shall next see, those who don't know you very well—who perhaps don't even know you at all—may be jumping to conclusions about your pregnancy and what it means.

7 Queen Bees, Flowerpots, Long-Lost Sisters

The visible physical fact of pregnancy frequently turns women into symbolic objects.

—ROBBIE E. DAVIS-FLOYD
Birth as an American Rite of Passage

By the seventh month of pregnancy my condition was, needless to say, blatantly obvious to anyone who looked my way. Indeed it was so obvious, so predominant, that I began to feel it was the pregnancy that people were seeing rather than the individual. Where once upon a time I'd mingle at parties and be asked much like anyone else in the room, "What do you do?" now I was asked, "When are you due?"

Clearly, I was no longer simply myself. I was an archetype, an icon, a Woman With Child. This redefinition proved a potent catalyst for change not only in the way that people viewed me, but in the way they treated me. And like most changes, it proved to be a mixed blessing.

Here is my most gratifying experience:

One day I had to make a trip to the Motor Vehicles Department to renew my driver's license. As anyone who lives in a heavily populated area will agree, the prospect of such an outing generally holds all the appeal of a cruise on the river Styx. The day I showed up, however, proved even more awful than usual. The computers, as the saying goes, "were down." I waited behind what seemed like several hundred people to accomplish the various bureaucratic tasks required to maintain my legal driver status. I got all my forms in order. I had a photo taken. Now it was time to pay the cashier, and yet another line snaked endlessly before me. Annoyed, I realized I would hardly have time to fulfill my quest. This was taking much longer than I'd bargained for and I had to get to my office to meet my first appointment. I motioned to a security guard to ask him if I could come back the next day without having to go through the entire rigmarole again.

"You are having a baby?" he asked.

("Bingo!" I thought.)

"Why, yes." I smiled sweetly.

Whereupon he gallantly ushered me to the head of the line.

Here is my most frustrating experience:

It happened to be during my seventh month that a new book of mine was published. In planning for the book's promotion its publisher had requested I undertake a fairly comprehensive publicity campaign, which would include TV appearances in several cities. As the publication date approached, I called the publisher's publicity department to ask about my itinerary.

"Oh," I was told, "our publicity director has decided to keep you at home and to arrange only press interviews."

"Only press?" I was astonished. I knew it would be detrimental to the book's success to narrow the scope of publicity so drastically. I pressed for a rationale, and after some embarrassed mumbling was told the publicity director did not believe it would be "appropriate" for me to do a televised book tour, my being in such a family way.

I couldn't believe my ears. What Neanderthal thinking! What about the precedent set by Jane Pauley, Joan Lunden, Katie Couric, and all the other women who had routinely appeared on camera in an advanced state of pregnancy? Besides, as I reminded my publisher, my book happened to be entirely related to family life. For Pete's sake, it was about marriage. What could be more appropriate, I asked, citing the old rhyme, "First come loves, then comes marriage, then comes so-and-so with a baby carriage!"

I prodded. I pestered. I won a partial victory. But I was—and I remain—peeved about the whole thing.

Well, as I said, being perceived as Woman With Child is a mixed bag. Sometimes people evidenced a kinder, gentler attitude toward me and made my day a little cheerier. Sometimes they offered up spontaneous "fringe benefits" (a seat on the bus, a helping hand with a cumbersome suitcase). But sometimes there was a condescension, or dismissiveness—as if my becoming more than myself had made me less than I was before.

When the pregnancy began, I wondered if I would be treated one particular way by men and another way by women as time advanced. But as it turned out, each gender evidenced a broad spectrum of responses. Some men were wildly solicitous; some charmingly chivalrous. Some men and women alike appeared determined to avoid me, seeming curiously unnerved by my condition. And some took an almost punitive approach. (The aforementioned publicity director, I am sad to say, was a woman.) Some women warmed my heart with their unconditional acceptance and made me feel as if I had, by virtue of my impending motherhood, gained entrance to a secret, exclusive sorority. Some (for reasons I would discover in time) seemed determined to scare me with "horror stories" of labor and birth.

Through it all, however, one truth stood out. Many people saw the pregnancy first, and me later, if at all. . . .

The Pregnant Woman as Rorschach Test

Linguist Deborah Tannen describes all members of the female gender as "marked."[1] By this she means that they are perceived as conveying a particular message by means of their appearance. A woman's clothing and accessories, her hairstyle, her makeup (or lack thereof) are all believed to "say something about her," and indeed evoke in others certain common associations.

I am sure no female is more "marked" than the pregnant woman.

Just about anyone who beholds a pregnant woman has some sort of reaction to the physical fact of her pregnancy. But what will that reaction be? It depends to some extent on cultural context, and even on when in the course of history this particular pregnancy is taking place (e.g., during an economic expansion or downturn, or during a time when conventional family life is considered fashionable or somewhat out of vogue). But in our heterogeneous contemporary society, where so many different people hold so many different kinds of values and priorities, it depends most of all on just who is doing the beholding.

In that sense, a pregnancy is like a kind of Rorschach test, the series of random inkblots which individuals interpret according to their predilections (where one may see a pair of lovers embracing, another may see soldiers locked in combat or perhaps only a couple of armchairs). Ultimately, the question is not "What does the image say?" but "What does it say about the people responding to it?"

Many factors may influence how any one person responds to the visible reality of a pregnant woman, including past personal experiences with conception and pregnancy, values concerning family life, ideas (pro or con) about women in the work force, conscious or unconscious conflicts involving sexuality, and even memories of how one felt if one's own mother became pregnant during one's childhood and gave birth to a sibling. Such memories, opinions, and associations, be they positive or negative, can all combine to create a sense of identification with the expectant mother or a sense of alienation from her. They may cause one individual to view a pregnant woman as a powerful goddess, while another views her as a fragile weakling, and still another as a walking time bomb.

Once a woman becomes pregnant, it doesn't take long for her to become only too aware that she has, by virtue of her pregnancy, become a "public property" of sorts. (Think of how many people assume it is fine and well to rub her tummy, as if she was some sort of carved ivory Buddha they might stroke for good luck.) As her condition becomes increasingly evident—and especially by the last trimester by which time it is almost certainly her most eye-catching physical characteristic—she is increasingly aware that she is serving as a canvas on which other people project their social suppositions, not to mention their private hopes and fears.

Of course, unlike the quintessential Rorschach blobs of ink, the pregnant woman has emotional responses to how other people feel about her. It is human nature to derive a part of how each of us feels about ourselves from how we believe others view us. So, it's difficult for her not to respond viscerally to the responses she engenders. What she finds she "symbolizes" to those around her on any given day may deeply affect her mood and her outlook.

Queen Bee

If one has no choice but to be a symbol, it is probably fair to say that most of us would find it nicest to be one that inspires something in the way of reverence, or at least respect. The good news: Many people find just such feelings awakened in them when they look at a woman who is with child.

In many primitive cultures, it was not uncommon for the pregnant woman to hold a place of honor among her peers. Deferred to and pampered by other women, prized by the proud papa and his kin, she was considered a most awe-inspiring entity, an object whose meaning and value transcended the interpersonal. She was the future personified, the Creative Force in action. She was the representation of health and abundance.

Certain perquisites went with this esteemed role of Queen Bee. The expectant mother got to partake in mystical rituals. She was lovingly inspected, fussed over, and good-naturedly teased. Moreover, she got to eat some of the choicest foodstuffs available.

Today, the Queen Bee persists as a pregnancy persona. Many people have only to look at a pregnant women to break into beaming smiles of approval. These smiles say, "You are worth cherishing," and the expectant mother may revel in their warmth.

The smiles sometimes emanate from other women, of course, and may signify a kind of "Atta girl" or "Been there too, Hon" message. But many pregnant women are amazed, and pleased, at how often the smiles emanate from men tuning in to their paternal or avuncular instincts.

> "I remember being very pregnant and waiting to meet my husband at a restaurant," recalled 29-year-old Sandra. "While I was waiting, I had to go to the bathroom. I realized, to my dismay, that this would mean walking past a long bar jammed with men who were acting pretty rowdy. Well, no choice, I had to go. But as I walked past the men they all turned and got these dopey, sweet looks on their faces and gave me the biggest grins. Normally, you walk through a bar and get leers. That day I felt the fatherhood in the room."

> "One day when I was in my last trimester," said 35-year-old Ester, "I was driving above the speed limit on a major highway where I know the police have a reputation for being very tough. I was pulled over by a fellow who looked like that state trooper in *Thelma and Louise.* I thought, 'I'm doomed.' He swaggered over to my car and asked for my license. While he was studying it, I remember making a little sound because the baby kicked really hard just then. The trooper looked down and at that point realized I was expecting. His entire demeanor changed. He asked if I was okay. He asked if I'd been hurrying to get to a hospital or to find a rest stop. I said, quite honestly, that no, I was just kind of in a hurry to get home and start dinner and hadn't been keeping an eye on the speedometer. You know, he *still* didn't give me a ticket. He asked me if this was my first kid, showed me a picture of his twin boys, told me to have a good, hearty dinner, and sent me on my way."

As in other cultures, preferential treatment is considered the Queen Bee's due. And though the perks are modernized, and usually involve small courtesies rather than grand fanfare, they serve the same function as always, in that they reinforce the perception that a pregnant woman is special.

In general, pregnant women—especially those who are far along enough to really appreciate the joys of, say, sitting down for the commute home, as opposed to standing up in a crowded aisle carrying a heavy briefcase—gladly and graciously accept whatever well-meant offerings come their way. It is hard to argue with goodwill.

Hard but not impossible.

For it must be said that some women react with suspicion when treated as Queen Bees. They worry about the possibility of Queen Bee backlash, i.e., that one person's innocent gesture of heartfelt respect may provide another person's excuse to discriminate against them. The bad news: That concern is not wholly unjustified.

Loose Cannons and Breakable Objects

Unfortunately, there are some people who view a pregnant woman as someone who is ipso facto weak or unreliable. More unfortunately still, such people are sometimes found in the pregnant woman's work milieu. At best, such individuals assume that an expectant mother's maternity mode will cause her to "lose her edge," whether she is a tax attorney or a taxi driver. At worst, they figure her condition has turned her into a proverbial bull in a china shop, a chaotic element apt to wreak all manner of havoc.

On the job, they may treat her as if she were in some way part of a handicapped group (perhaps perceived as the "hormonally challenged") which, while entitled to supposedly equal treatment under the law, is nevertheless the victim of subtle but significant prejudice.

"Throughout my pregnancy, I seemed to be getting fewer and fewer choice assignments," recalls Lauren, a 28-year-old reporter for a metropolitan section of a large urban daily newspaper. "I went from routinely covering breaking news and important stories on issues like crime and local politics to what I call 'fluff stuff,' things like the local tulip festival and new cubs at the zoo. I asked the assignment editors about it. One said I was imagining things. Another admitted I was right, but felt that I should—and I quote— just take it easy while I was baking my bun.''

Some women felt their bosses or coworkers not only had a view of them as Loose Cannons or Breakable Objects, but that these people virtually counted on the fact that everyone else would share their particular stereotypical view.

"The most infuriating episode for me," said 35-year-old Martha, a successful tax accountant, "was when I was seven or eight months pregnant. A partner in my firm suggested I take over a particular audit because the IRS agent on the case was known to be very tough to deal with. The partner said, 'Alright, look, you go in there looking haggard, you bite your lip a little, you look real upset, maybe you start to cry. How hard is he going to be if he thinks you might go into premature labor right on his desk?'

"Oh, well. I suppose I should have laughed. As obnoxious as this comment was, at least it meant I was assumed to have some usefulness. I've heard worse stories."

There are worse stories, indeed. Some where women are passed over for promotions. Some where they lose their jobs altogether. Some where the level of insensitivity in the workplace runs so blatantly high that pregnant women are themselves tempted to quit.

Should anyone reading this be thinking of jumping to the conclusion that most of those who discriminate against expectant mothers are men, think again. As the *Wall Street Journal,* citing recent research, has reported, "Women managers are responsible for much of the pregnancy discrimination at work."[2]

At first it may be hard to fathom why this is so. But women may have all kinds of rationales for behaving badly toward their pregnant subordinates. Some may feel fearful of superiors frowning on them should they display any special treatment toward expectant mothers, so they go 180 degrees in the other direction. Some may have had unpleasant work-related experiences during their own pregnancies, and perhaps feel, "If I could handle it, so should you."

Whatever the reasons behind it, being viewed as Loose Cannons or Breakable Objects is often tough on pregnant women even if it doesn't ultimately result in a demotion or a firing. It may make them want to conceal their conditions as long as possible, even if that means dressing in a highly uncomfortable, impractical manner. It may also make them loathe to admit, even to themselves, when they feel fatigued. Afraid of being ostracized, they may keep going long past the time when common sense tells them to take a break. For to admit to experiencing any pregnancy symptoms may feel to them like an admission of inadequacy.

Even though whatever job they may have is now one of two jobs (the second being the production of a healthy baby), they hardly seek to take credit for this feat. In fact they may do just the opposite, overcompensating in Job Number One and making light of Job Number Two. Ironically, this "just ignore my pregnancy" demeanor can itself reinforce yet another negative pregnancy stereotype . . .

The Pregnant Woman as a Flowerpot

Some women's rights advocates have begun to popularize a phrase—and find fault with a concept—they call the "flowerpot theory of pregnancy." First coined by Caroline Whitbeck, it refers to a viewpoint of human procreation that maintains, in effect, the man plants a seed, the woman houses it, and, poof, it comes out a baby.[3] Rather than equating the woman with the nurturing soil, water, and sun's energy, this philosophy equates her with a kind of benign container, nothing more.

Those who see a pregnant woman as a Flowerpot believe she should have no special consideration whatsoever. They neither fuss over her nor ostracize her. On the job they regard her condition the same as any medical condition that might lead to a brief absence from work. Other than allowing for that absence, they look at her blankly if she maintains that there are perhaps certain duties she ought not perform at this time.

One would think that, on the face of it, this might satisfy any woman who was concerned with being discriminated against. But some women believe that to treat a pregnancy like a case of shingles, a sprained ankle, or anything else requiring only some brief recuperation time is actually itself discriminatory.

Pregnancy, many women's rights advocates argue, is *sui generis,* a thing unto itself. As sociologist Barbara Rothman has asked, "How can uniqueness be made to fit into an equality mode?"[4]

This may sound to some like a case of feminists wanting their cake and eating it too, but Rothman's question bears thinking about. And the solution will not make itself easily known, for as Rothman notes, "The liberal argument, the fairness argument, the equal rights argument, these all break down when we look at women who are, or are becoming, mothers."[5]

It is not possible in this book to sort out the complex issues of what, exactly, is fair and just when it comes to a pregnant woman's rights under the law, but one thing can be said here with certainty: Pregnant women often feel irritated, even belittled, when they are viewed as mere Flowerpots.

"I remember being pregnant," said Allison, a chef for a catering company who was pregnant with her first child at age 32, "and my boss asked me to make up some smoked fish platters. I smelled the fish and just about passed out. I said, 'Listen George, I am really sorry. I can't seem to deal with smoked fish today. I'll get someone else to do it.' I mean there was no way I was going to be able deal with this without losing my lunch and ruining our client's lunch. But he looked at me blankly—like, what's your problem. Even when I explained about my nausea, he looked blank. It wasn't that he didn't understand. I knew his wife, and she'd had four kids. I think he just couldn't equate 'employee' with 'pregnant' so he chose to ignore it."

Of course pregnant women may be treated as Flowerpots not only in the workplace, but outside of it. And those who treat them as such are certainly not always men:

"I was pregnant with my second child," recalls 31-year-old Cindy, "and I was riding Amtrak to Washington, D.C., on business. I got on at Philadelphia and sat next to a semi-elderly lady. When she was getting ready to get off the train at Baltimore she stood up and said, 'Excuse me, dear, would you mind getting that for me?' She pointed to a large, overstuffed bag in the overhead luggage rack. I thought, well maybe she doesn't know I'm pregnant. But, believe me, I was so far gone you couldn't miss it. Either I was expecting or I had swallowed a watermelon whole. I really was taken aback, but I managed to say, 'I'm so sorry, but I'd have to stand on the seat to reach it and I'm afraid I'll fall.' She rolled her eyes, like I was out of my mind, or maybe just a wimp, but finally asked someone else for assistance."

It can be maddening indeed for a pregnant woman to be considered a Flowerpot. For that implies that whoever does so— whether for some self-serving reason, or out of a misguided attempt to be "fair"—is choosing to disregard the momentous task in which she is involved. It implies also that further problems may lie around the bend. Because by logical extension, people who don't give a woman credit for being pregnant will hardly give her credit for being a mother.

The Invisible Woman

Believe it or not, there is yet another way an expectant mother may be treated which can be at least as unnerving, if not more so, than the Flowerpot response. That is when people go out of their way to ignore her altogether. They neglect to acknowledge not just her condition, but her very existence.

The more a pregnancy becomes visible, the more some people may treat an expectant mother like a cipher, a nonentity. Sometimes this affects one's professional dealings:

"When my pregnancy became obvious, people stopped coming to me with new project ideas," said 34-year-old Casey, who coheads a Los Angeles based TV production company. "People who had long worked primarily with me now directed their comments to my partner, as though I weren't even in the room. I don't know if they thought my brain cells had atrophied or if I was going to take my baby and retire to a cave, or what!"

And sometimes it affects one's personal life:

"For a long time I tried to get pregnant," said 41-year-old Rita. "And many of my friends were in the same boat, having put off childbearing until relatively late in life. While I was doing the whole fertility regime, some of these friends wanted to commiserate with me every step of the way. But once I actually became pregnant, several of them began to distance themselves from me. It wasn't very subtle the way they did it. They just stopped calling, and even when we were together at some party or function, they made obligatory small talk and then found some excuse to turn away."

As lamentable as these stories are, they are, alas, not altogether uncommon. The reasons why some people may treat expectant mothers as Invisible Women are myriad.

If they have come to rely on her in a professional or personal sense, they may experience themselves as being abandoned by the expectant mother, and worry that she will no longer pay attention to them or "take care" of them the way she used to. Deep down, they may even fear that her pregnancy will cause something unfortunate to befall her and that she may be damaged or even face death. Rather than contend with such feelings, they avoid her.

If they themselves would like to carry children in their bodies but cannot (and this may apply as equally to some frustrated members of the male gender as it does to some women with fertility obstacles), they may experience palpable envy of her circumstance. Rather than own up to their envy, they withdraw.

Avoidance and withdrawal can also take place when someone is burdened with unhappy memories of that person's own pregnancy or that of a loved one (perhaps a wife or the person's own mother), when someone feels awkward about sexual matters (perhaps he or she doesn't feel comfortable with the knowledge that a pregnant woman has had to have sex in order to get that way), and when the entire idea of pregnancy and family life is anathema (perhaps the person has chosen a different way of life and feels somewhat defensive about that choice).

Finally, and in a broader sense, it has been suggested by cultural anthropologist Robbie E. Davis-Floyd that in our contemporary society, some people, to one degree or another, feel put off by the pregnant woman because she is a "walking representative of nature in a culture that seeks to deny nature's power."[6]

In each of these instances, it appears that what we have is a shunning of the expectant mother by people who, rather than face their own feelings and fears, choose not to face her.

The Secret Sorority

Most expectant mothers I spoke with agreed that gender was not the primary factor which determined whether any given individual perceived them and treated them as Queen Bees, Loose Cannons, Flowerpots, or Invisible Women during the course of their pregnancies. However, there is one very pronounced female-only phenomenon of perception which frequently occurs. A great many mothers-to-be commented on the vast numbers of mothers-already who suddenly treated them as some sort of Long Lost Sisters and who seemed to invite them—through winks and smiles, through confidences, comradely squeezes and claps on the shoulder—to join a kind of de facto secret sorority.

This sudden acceptance often generates in a pregnant woman reciprocal feelings of warmth and intimacy. Her newfound sisterhood can be a great source of strength and joy, and can make her feel quite heady, especially initially.

> "I felt like I'd entered this new world," said 26-year-old Maria. "It was glorious making so many deep connections with women who may have been somewhat reserved before. Suddenly, women were confiding in me. Even my straightlaced great-aunts were telling me earthy stories."

❖

"There were so many advantages to being in this club," recalled 28-year-old Jessie. "When I had any little aches or pains, there seemed always to be someone to turn to who would say, 'Oh, yes. That happened to me.' When I felt blah, sort of fat and frumpy, it helped me remember to be proud. When I felt like I was on a roller coaster ride, having given my body over to this baby, I remembered this pregnancy was earning me a badge of honor as a female."

Often, women pregnant for the first time express surprise at the existence of the secret sorority of motherhood. Though they are, for the most part, pleased with their newfound roles of Long Lost Sisters, they wonder: *How on earth could I have been around so long and not even known that this club existed?* The fact is pregnancy is one of those special life experiences, like orgasmic sex or romantic love, that one simply has to live through before fully comprehending. No amount of voyeurism or secondhand knowledge will suffice. Once women have undergone this pregnancy rite of passage it is only natural that they show a high level of interest in new initiates. At the same time, of course, initiates are extremely interested in pregnancy "veterans," which serves to cement the new bond.

As Maria and Jessie pointed out, the advantages that come with entering the sisterhood are numerous. Self-doubts may be assuaged, self-esteem may be enhanced, intimate affiliations may be made in a frenetic world where such associations are increasingly difficult to come by. Moreover, once in the sorority, one has access to a network of people who can be called day or night with questions and concerns that may seem too personal or not serious enough to address to a medical professional.

It's easy to understand why, overall, joining the sisterhood is experienced by most pregnant women as a positive part of their pregnancies, in many ways a genuine privilege. But even the best of experiences may have its downsides, and there are one or two that expectant mothers tend to mention with relation to their new "club."

One is that there are times when advice seems almost too plentiful. It's one thing to ask questions and get welcome information in return. It's another to feel a bit smothered by sisters who sometimes seem a shade too eager to impart every detail of their wisdom at every conceivable opportunity. (I myself recall a stint of real-estate shopping where a zealous new mother took time out from showing her house to pull me aside and instruct me as to how to prepare my nipples for nursing.)

Such impromptu attempts to be of assistance and to forge a bond, generally well-meant though they are, can be somewhat startling and a bit off-putting, but they are nowhere near as disconcerting as the second dubious distinction of the sisterhood, i.e., the sharing of what I have come to think of as Terror Tales From the Labor Room.

Many pregnant women comment with great consternation on what they consider the distressing and peculiar phenomenon of birthgiving alumni who feel compelled to impart to mothers-to-be every graphic detail of every pain, complaint, or complication that made them unhappy or uncomfortable during labor and delivery. Cornered at parties, in rest rooms, or on line at the automated teller machine, pregnant women seem to hear no end of unsolicited terror tales. Some are related conspiratorially. ("Probably no one's told you about the hemorrhoids, so let me.") Some include implicit or explicit warnings. ("I said no to the epidural and felt like a Mack truck ran over my genitals.") At times, the tales tend to take on mythic proportions. ("My baby had the biggest head circumference ever recorded at my hospital.")

Expectant mothers, who are already anxious about the prospect of facing so great a challenge as giving birth, tend not only to be somewhat intimidated but profoundly perplexed by such narratives. What on earth can these sisters be thinking? Are they trying to frighten them? Are they trying to undermine their confidence? Are they putting them through some sort of hazing ritual that comes with joining the motherhood sorority?

Actually the answer is generally none of the above. In fact, the stories serve a therapeutic purpose for the women telling them. They are the equivalent of both modern macho locker-room tales and of ancient male battle lore (where the person with the "worst" story is perceived as the most powerful). They are a woman's way of saying, "I got the ball past that sonovabitch linebacker"; "I scaled the mountain during a terrible storm"; "I stared the dragon in the eye and lived to tell."

The terror tales are a woman's way of processing her awesome experience and the emotions that went along with that experience. Certainly, imparting these tales to expectant mothers may at times be inappropriate. Often the talebearer herself knows this, and may follow up her saga with a sheepish "Oops, I guess I shouldn't have said that to you." But to whom else would she or could she say it?

Sadly, our society has to date provided precious few forums in which a woman can discuss her childbirth so that it makes sense to her. Nevertheless, she needs to process the many events and emotions which comprised it so that they begin to form some kind of cohesive whole. She may feel the need to justify her choices, or to lament them. She may need to express triumph, or to mourn. And she will surely need to begin the healing process if emotional wounds resulted from labor and delivery, whether from a traumatic physical circumstance, from unsympathetic treatment from someone in attendance at the birth, or from the fact that some aspect of the birth experience was incongruent with her expectations.

Until and unless such forums become an integral part of postpartum care for all women, as they most certainly should, childbirth veterans are destined to roam cocktail parties and supermarket aisles in the style of the Ancient Mariner, searching for someone with whom to share their stories.

In the meanwhile, however, it is wise to adopt a strategy which will allow you to cope with other women's forbidding labor and delivery tales. Like most women, you don't want to offend your newfound sisters, who after all have so much of value to offer you. But at the same time, you don't want to be unduly influenced by any negative aspects of their experience.

Learning what to take in and what not to take in from the outside is, in more ways than one, critical during pregnancy. On a physical level, one needs to take in good nourishment and keep out the "junk." On an interpersonal level, one needs to let in the support and to try to detach from messages or projections that feel toxic.

❖ AN EXPECTANT MOTHER'S PRIVILEGES AND PREROGATIVES

Remember, the way people "type" you when you're a pregnant woman is a reflection on them, *not you.* Like it or not, people are apt to project all manner of things onto you when you are expecting, some very negative. However, once you accept that unhappy or inappropriate responses individuals have to pregnancy are about their conflicts, you can resist internalizing negative projections that come your way. If someone treats you in an unpleasant fashion, odds are that person has an unpleasant association with pregnancy for reasons you may never know. Agreed, it sometimes seems as if such people are acting out of petty motives, or that they are simply being jerks. Go ahead and feel angry. There's nothing wrong with that. And by all means stand up for your rights when necessary. Just don't buy into their baggage. Don't let them dictate to you how to define yourself.

Be prepared to experience multiple personas. Another facet to being a Rorschach test is that different people can see different things in you *simultaneously.* So don't be surprised if you are "assigned," say, one role by your family, another by coworkers, a third by your single girlfriends, and yet another by women who are mothers themselves. In the course of one day, you may well have to react and respond to all of these perceptions, and it can certainly get to be emotionally confusing. It helps to remember that *your* central sense of yourself is the one that counts. Stay focused on your values and your priorities. (Remember why you decided to have a child in the first place and go from there.) And whatever else you do, hang on to your sense of humor. It's essential.

Relish your Queenlike moments. For many, the predominant association to pregnancy is positive. If a majority of people seem to instinctively treat women like Queen Bees, perhaps Nature planned it thus. If pregnancy weren't, at least in some ways, rewarded on a sociocultural level, our species probably would have died out long ago.

Don't fight Mother Nature on this one. If assistance is offered in a sincere and gracious manner, try to accept it graciously. And don't be too proud to ask for help if you need it.

Think you're undeserving of royal status? Not a chance. Whatever your occupation—brain surgeon, CPA, secretary, homemaker—you are moonlighting while pregnant, devoting energy to growing an extraordinarily complex being. Your efforts merit acknowledgment.

Besides, your reign won't last forever. Once the baby arrives, he or she will be Center of Attention and Ruler of the Household for quite some time to come. So enjoy your tenure as Queen Bee while you can.

Remember, being pregnant is tantamount to hanging a sign on your head saying "Give Me Advice." No matter what, as an expectant mother, you are bound to receive counsel from practically every woman who has ever had the pregnancy and mothering experience. Open season has been declared, and you just have to live with that. But, and this is a big but, you are entitled to put appropriate boundaries around the advice that comes your way. Rehearse some "comebacks" that will serve you when you'd otherwise be at a loss. Practice saying, "OK, thanks, but I want to figure this out on my own," or, "Isn't that interesting. I'm glad that worked for you," or simply, "My, look at the time. I've got to fly!"

Raise your shield when you hear terror tales. The visualization technique already described in the second chapter of this book—wherein you imagine yourself and your baby contained in a bubble of cleansing light which repels negativity—may well prove useful to you when faced with a sister imparting a birth tale that makes you uneasy. Remember that inside this benign space no harm can befall you. In addition, counter any frightening or unsettling communications by silently repeating positive affirmations to yourself. Practice thinking, "I feel sorry that this person had this experience. But this is not my experience." If what is coming your way is not helpful to you, detach from it.

Plan and enjoy "retreat time." What with all the attention (positive or negative), all the advice, and all the tales you'll be told, you may well feel like your psychic space is being invaded. To compensate for this, don't neglect to plan and enjoy time in physical and emotional circumstances that feel safe to you. Curl up in a favorite armchair, read your favorite authors. Roll up the windows and play music you love on your car stereo. Revisit a cozy, intimate restaurant with your spouse. Plan time with your most dear and trusted friends.

Pregnancy, especially the later months, is a good time to burrow in and hunker down. Take whatever time you need to regroup right now, for you are entering the final innings.

8 Home Stretch

We must seek bodies for our children.

—OSAGE INDIAN CHANT

"*Rubber baby buggy bumpers, rubber baby buggy bumpers . . .*" *Eight months pregnant, and the childhood tongue twister circled through my mind as I scavenged through my local kiddie-equipment-and-clothing emporium trying to make ready for my newborn. Nodding at fellow package-laden mothers-to-be swaying down the crowded aisles, I eyed infant doodads and whatchamacallits, feeling half purposeful, half dazed. The shopping list of "must-haves" my sister-in-law, mother of two, graciously compiled for my benefit seemed endless: stroller, rocking chair, crib, car seat, changing table, baby carrier, baby monitor, stretchies, booties (and endless other little teeny "-ies"), liquid aspirin substitute, calamine lotion, syrup of ipecac for accidental poisoning (Oh, God, did she say poisoning?).*

Somehow I managed to procure an armload of paraphernalia and place another order for delivery. But later, contemplating my many purchases, I worried about lead-based paints and sharp edges. Had I thoroughly checked for these and other hazards? What if an oversight of mine should lead to some horrible mishap? I'd never forgive myself. And my mother, whose sole hope of grandmother-hood lay with me, her only daughter (who had put this off long enough, thank you very much), would have my head on a platter.

Later that week the deliveries arrived, and that night I wandered the hallways of our new house and inventoried the goods. In the moonlight, a bassinet cast an oblong shadow on the nursery wall. Nursery? Bassinet? I stared at the ruffle-covered cradle, trying to imagine a baby, an actual baby, nestled inside. In a way, the idea of an infant coming to live with us seemed as plausible as the Three Bears dropping in for porridge. But then my nightgown began jumping up and down. The baby seemed to be prac-ticing his break dancing routine, and reality became undeni-able once more.

It was going to happen, wasn't it? That's why I bought all this merchandise. That's why my husband and I had begun spending every Tuesday night at a childbirth class, sitting on pillows, practicing relaxation techniques, and asking ques-tions like "How, exactly, do you know when it's time to go to the hospital?"

Tuesday night, I thought, hmmm. That reminded me . . . something about Tuesday night. Oh, yes. Snatching a wisp of a detail that almost got away from me, I made a mental note to remind my husband that this week's class was switched to Wednesday. On second thought, I decided to write it down and stick a Post-it note on the bathroom mirror where I'd be sure not to miss it. I added the note CLASS WED to a cluster of others: CLEANER PICKUP; VIDEO RETURN; CALL PLUMBER. Lately, I'd been so absentminded, I'd forgotten my credit card at the baby emporium and lost an automated bank card and a set of car keys in the past two weeks. I'd have forgotten my feet if they weren't attached. Come to think of it, I mused staring down at my stomach, I couldn't see my feet anymore. I could only presume they were where I last spotted them.

Big as Life

By the eighth month of pregnancy things loom large. Take one's profile, for example. On a woman's outside, there are astoundingly hefty breasts, puffy ankles, a rotund tummy—skin stretched so taut across it that it itches. Inside, there are squashed lungs and squished intestines (leading to a cacophony of gassy emissions), and a bladder more crowded than a ladies' room at intermission. All organs are pushed aside to make way for the Amazing Expanding Baby, whose completely formed body is now adding fat reserves along with assorted finishing touches.

But the physical dimension is not the only one in which things weigh heavily. In the emotional dimension, what seems to be growing larger and larger every day is the Inevitability Factor. The baby which began to seem more vivid and viable when quickening began, is exponentially more of a reality now. And that reality brings with it a list of deadlines.

It's time to address with speed and seriousness anything one may have been putting off—arranging a maternity leave from work, thinking about who will help out during the first weeks the baby's at home, focusing on a post-baby budget, and the like. It is also time to start taking responsibility for deciding on some fundamental details, like figuring out what accoutrements and accessories the new little resident in one's home will require.

In generations gone by, creating the ideal environment for baby was not afforded the kind of premeditation it is today. In great-grandmother's era, people considered themselves lucky if they could locate a space that wasn't already occupied by another member of the household. But, face it, this is a thoroughly modern infant you're bearing, and it needs *stuff*. Lots of stuff. And it needs a space of its own in which to feel warm and cozy, safe and appropriately stimulated.

A pregnant woman in her late stages is generally itching to start preparing that space and collecting that long list of baby gadgets. No more dawdling, no more kidding around. It is time to build a nest. And she wants to do it *now*!

Nesting Fever

The zeal with which a pregnant woman organizes and orchestrates a place for baby in the later phases of the third trimester is a well-known phenomenon. Mention it to any new father and he will probably shake his head in awe and amazement in recalling how much energy his wife was able to manifest, in spite of an unwieldy load which the uninitiated might assume would generate awkwardness and lethargy. But nesting fever is yet another typical pregnancy experience which seems to be precipitated by both the body and the mind.

On a physical level, the pregnant woman whose baby has dropped deep down into the pelvic cavity (as typically happens, at least with first-time mothers, by four weeks or so before the due date) can literally get a "second wind" when pressure on her diaphragm is relieved. As a result of the dropping, which is also referred to as *lightening* (a good word for it), she may feel more pep than she's felt in a while, and instinctively take advantage of this little window of opportunity which Mother Nature has afforded her.

On an emotional level, there is also a very good reason for nesting fever. For perfectly understandable reasons, various anxieties—some of which may have arisen earlier in the pregnancy but been temporarily suppressed—are reactivated as the due date draws near. Focusing intensively on the minutiae of nest preparation offers the psyche a convenient way of avoiding the kind of anxiety overload that might accompany inactivity.

Rather than dwell on, say, how—or how soon, or indeed whether—she will return to work after the birth, a pregnant woman with the nesting bug can dwell on the competing advantages of Mickey Mouse versus Peter Rabbit decor. Rather than obsessing on the several hundred thousand dollars it will, all told, cost to raise a child from infancy to adulthood in America today, she can debate the wisdom of springing for the car seat with the removable, washable liner and the quick-fasten safety buckle. Rather than court the terror that can accompany such thoughts as "Having this baby means the end of my life as I know it!" she can find solace in thinking about how happy her baby will be in the space she has lovingly readied.

For many women, extra-ambitious nesting temporarily imparts a sense of control. Having virtually no say-so in such fundamental issues as when her baby will show up and what sort of temperament it will be endowed with from the start—and less control than she would like over the myriad ways in which her newborn will impact her personal and professional life—a mother-to-be may pull out all the stops when it comes to making her nest *just so*.

She may devote herself tirelessly to poring over paint samples and wallpaper swatches. She may even decide, against her husband's objections and her mother's impassioned pleas on behalf of restraint, to paint or paper the nursery herself. She may brood endlessly over selecting just the right curtains or perhaps try making them. She may arrange furniture, rearrange it, fluff, dust, and move it all back to where it was in the first place. And even if she is of the mind that it is better not to tempt fate by actually bringing baby furniture into her home before the baby's birth (as a number of women are) she may perform these same chores over and over, indefatigably, in her mind. In short, she may display superhuman strength and stamina as she readies her nest for its precious new occupant.

The belief (often only a semiconscious one) that underlies such Herculean feats is often: "If I can do all this, I can do it all. Motherhood is perfectly manageable, and I shall manage it perfectly." Ironically enough, though, the nesting process itself can present confounding conundrums, offering even the most single-minded, perfectionist nest-builder glimpses into her uncertain and vaguely chaotic future.

The Tip of the Iceberg

In our consumer-oriented society, a large part of the nesting process involves the purchasing of items aimed at making life with baby as pleasant and easy as possible. But the dizzying array of options can be overwhelming. And each choice can open a Pandora's box of woes.

One would think that tackling the basics (something for the

baby to sleep in, for example, or bottles for milk) would be easy. But alas, nothing is as simple as it seems.

Take, for example, the saga of a 32-year-old first-time mother, Tina, who set herself the mission of purchasing a crib:

"I told some friends that my husband and I were going crib shopping come the weekend. I thought they'd say, 'Oh, how nice.' Instead they all started sermons that began with the words, 'Make sure . . .' 'Make sure you get high railings so he can't climb over when he starts to stand up.' 'Make sure the bars aren't too far apart or he'll get his head caught and strangle himself.' 'Make sure you get the kind that turns into a junior bed or you'll be throwing your money away.'

"That wasn't all. One of my friends gave me a big speech about how I shouldn't have a crib at all and how my child would grow up insecure and neurotic unless we let him sleep in a family bed with us. I felt instantly guilty. Was it cruel to buy a crib?

"My husband tried to jolly me out of it. He promised that we would consider trying a family bed, but reminded me that the kid would still need a place to nap—unless the whole family was going to take a siesta every afternoon. So we went crib hunting. And we ran into a salesman who tried to sell us some two-thousand-dollar contraption that vibrated all night long. Not only did he lead us to believe the baby would never sleep through the night without it, but that if we got it, he would develop a superior intellect and a serene demeanor. Kind of a cross between Gandhi and Einstein. He all but promised early admission to Yale."

Despite friends' admonitions and salesmen's pitches, Tina and her husband bought an unpretentious wooden crib which neither vibrated nor levitated nor converted into a wall unit or a Chippendale table. (They did *make sure* it had an adjustable railing and met all current federal safety standards.) But the entire episode turned out to be more of a psychological ordeal than anticipated.

Twenty-eight-year-old Maxine ran into a somewhat similar dilemma when she decided it was time to lay in a supply of bottles and nipples.

"You would think," she lamented, "that buying these things would be relatively unchallenging. But then you start looking and you see that some bottles aren't really bottles, but sort of plastic tubes that you line with disposable bags. I wondered if that was environmentally correct. It sure seemed easier than sterilizing bottles, but I didn't want to be chastised for it. As for nipples, that was a whole other story. My sister said I should get these nipples that are supposed to be orthodontically correct. My coworker said to be sure to get the kind that are most like real nipples so the baby wouldn't get confused when I went back to work and left my expressed breast milk. I thought, 'Of course the baby will be confused. I'm confused!' I didn't even know if I really wanted to breast-feed or not, but everyone sort of assumed I would, so I ended up buying the Mommylike nipples and the bottles that were supposed to be good for storing breast milk and so on. Talk about pressure. I remember standing at the checkout counter hoping that nothing I'd bought would 'give me away' as a potential bad mother."

For Tina and Maxine, and countless other women, buying baby supplies brought them face-to-face with profoundly emotional decisions. They wondered, should they share their beds with their children? (And if they do how will it affect the children's psyches for good or ill? What's more, how on earth will it affect their marriages?) Will they breast-feed? (And if so will they nurse exclusively, and for how long? How will they be able to add this enormous commitment to all their others?)

The answers, needless to say, are hard to fathom. The baby isn't born yet, and what may be envisioned is limited. Adopting a unilateral policy, no matter how advanced a pregnancy may be, is like trying to steer around an iceberg without taking into account how much of it lies out of view. The mother-to-be can, and should, read books about such matters as the pros and cons of family beds and breast-feeding. She can go to La Leche meetings, ask lots of questions, and see what she thinks. She can, in general, gather as much information as possible and plan accordingly. However (and this is a very large however), she finally must accept that any decision she makes pre-baby may well change post-baby when idealism collides head-on with realism and when she will be faced with the moment-to-moment imperative to do *whatever works*.

The same applies when it comes to factoring in matters of political correctness—another contemporary bugaboo that tends to plague nesting mothers. Laying in her supplies, a woman can't help but wonder: Will disposable bottles mark her as a playground pariah? And if that's the case, what about disposable diapers? The truth is she will not know all there is to know about her needs and her baby's habits until later. For now, she might do well to leave her options open, perhaps buying a little of this and little of that to try.

Then, of course, there is the issue of status to consider. What kind of stroller ought she purchase? Are those ones with the Italian-sounding brand names really all they're cracked up to be? And even if they're not, is it important for her to have one anyway so that when she wheels her child to the A&P everyone will think she knows what she's doing? And what about those itty-bitty Christian Dior all-in-ones that look so very precious and cost so very much? Don't infants grow out of them in about six seconds? But wouldn't she like just a couple anyway for when the relatives come to coo? No!? What's wrong with her? Is she being too practical?

Pandora's decision-making demons seem endless. But, as they myth tells us, the last thing out of the box is a salvation—hope. For the mothers-to-be, there's always this hope: that some baby-related status symbols and trendy developmental gizmos and perhaps even a few basic necessities will be "showered" upon her when friends and family converge for the party that officially welcomes her to the parenting club. In fact, by the end of her baby shower she may be up to her earlobes in musical mobiles, black-and-white flash cards, white noise machines, designer footie pajamas, and hooded terry towels.

Perhaps her nearest and dearest have even chipped in for the super deluxe stroller she secretly yearned for but couldn't quite justify. Or perhaps they've preempted her agonizing over the diaper dilemma by treating her to—depending on their own convictions—a year's subscription to a diaper service or a half truckload full of Pampers.

Any or all of this can take some of the pressure off. But, shower or no, nesting decisions can be daunting if an expectant mother imagines she can figure out all the ins and outs of mothering ahead of time, and if she believes creating a perfectly appointed nursery will obliterate all her doubts and fears.

Approached with the right attitude—one which says, "Hey, this is fun and helps take my mind off my worries a bit"—nesting fever is a marvelous diversion. If you are caught in its throes, enjoy it as much as you can. Approached as a relentless obsessive quest, however, nesting will end up being a burden, proving *too much* of a distraction for your own good at a time when other important deadlines loom.

The most obvious of all: The baby, growing ever larger, can't stay inside forever. One day, one day soon, it's going to have to come out. It's entirely reasonable for a mother-to-be to be somewhat preoccupied with how she will deal with that momentous passage.

Choosing a Childbirth Class

Happily, a structure exists to provide at least some inkling of an answer. Today prepared childbirth courses are routinely attended by vast numbers of pregnant women (first-timers most frequently, though refresher courses are not uncommon). But, once again, informed choices must be made.

As most women who have reached their third trimester are probably aware, there are myriad options available today in addition to the ubiquitous Lamaze class. There are Bradley classes, which focus on deep relaxation rather than Lamaze sequenced breathing techniques. And there are classes that teach a combination of Bradley and Lamaze techniques. There are also cropping up increasing numbers of classes promising instruction in so-called "painless childbirth," "spiritual childbirth," "holistic birth," and the like. What are the differences? And how can an expectant mother know which will be the most comfortable for her?

Perri Klass, the physician who wrote of bearing a child in

medical school, also wrote of her experience with childbirth education during her pregnancy, and summarized one key difference in approach. Describing her experience with her initial choice, a class given at her hospital, she wrote: "At the first meeting it became clear that the class's major purpose was in preparing people to be good patients. . . . The teacher exposed us to various procedures so we would cooperate properly when they were performed on us. Asked whether a given procedure was necessary she said that was up to our doctor."[1]

Klass was underwhelmed with this manner of instruction and transferred to a childbirth class that met at a local day-care center. "This class," she wrote, "if anything, designed to teach people how to be 'bad patients.' The teacher explained the pros and cons of the various interventions, and we discussed under what circumstances we might or might not accept them."[2]

Klass is not the only one to comment on the distinction between obedience and disobedience classes. A number of women I talked with were disappointed after signing up for classes at their hospitals or doctors' offices. They'd imagined they would spend most of the time learning how to help manage their contractions and otherwise take an active role in their children's birth, but found instead that while they were given some instruction of that nature, the bulk of the class time was spent explaining what was going to be done *to* them during the labor and delivery process.

Of course, if after giving the matter due consideration, a woman decides a hi-tech birth is definitely what she wants, this sort of general familiarization with the "standard operating procedure" may be all she is interested in. That, of course, is her prerogative. However, any woman who wants to keep her options open would do well to select a childbirth education forum which offers instruction in being, if not a "bad patient," at least a participatory one who is oriented to saying "yes" or "no" to any given medical intervention based on its benefits versus its risks.

If she sets out to find such a course, she must exercise good sense in finding a class that suits her desires. And she should beware generalizations about what sort of instruction to sign on for. What she'll probably discover, if she asks around, is a general belief among like-minded women that Bradley classes (named for founder Dr. Robert Bradley, who developed his method of natural childbirth from watching animals deliver their young) offer a more "disobedient" perspective than the more widely accepted Lamaze instruction. But it would be wrong to assume that all instructors who teach Lamaze techniques wholly endorse—or encourage their students to unquestioningly accept—the high-tech system, even if they have opted to work more or less within it. (By the way, though Lamaze has come to be thought of by some as "conventional" or "conservative," it should be noted that it is thanks to the persistence of early Lamaze instructors that general anesthesia has been eliminated as a standard childbirth intervention and that fathers are routinely admitted into the delivery room.)

Likewise, it would be wrong to assume that teachers of alternative methods to Lamaze are any less likely to foist a particular agenda upon pregnant women than the most dyed-in-the-wool supporter of the hi-tech system. Regardless of how "spiritual" or "holistic" an instructor claims to be, expectant mothers must be wary of grandiose claims, such as the promise of pain-free childbirth or a guarantee that one will see angels between contractions. Expecting childbirth without some attendant pain is like expecting to freeze water without getting ice. And while angels may indeed be present at each and every birth, a laboring woman will generally find herself too preoccupied to give them the once-over even if they should drop their cloaks of invisibility.

When it comes to finding a class that teaches you to become a savvy and self-assertive birthgiver, while at the same time not building up unrealistic expectations, the safest bet is to speak directly with individual instructors whose courses you may be considering. Ascertain if there is a rigid dogma attached to the class (if there is, it's probably a good one to pass by). Ask where the class is given (if it's at a particular institution, such as a hospital, it's more likely to echo the belief system of that institution than if it is given at an instructor's home or on some other type of neutral ground). Ask about class size (a very large class may not allow time for addressing individual concerns or special circumstances). And make certain whatever class you're considering integrates your spouse in a way in which he feels comfortable.

You might consider investigating not only single method classes, but classes where instructors take an integrated approach, teaching, for example, Bradley-style deep relaxation and Lamaze-style breathing (integration pretty much ensures the absence of inflexible dogma, and one never knows exactly what will come in handy). And you might want to take into account whether any class time is devoted to basic infant care instruction and postpartum discussions (because birthing a baby, as intimidating as that may be, may not feel half as intimidating as figuring out what to do with the child when he or she shows up).

No matter how well and how thoughtfully one chooses a childbirth class, of course, when it finally comes down to it no one can teach a woman how to give birth. Childbirth is one of those things that simply has to be lived through and dealt with in the moment. But taking a prepared childbirth course serves other invaluable functions as well. For one thing, such classes offer an expectant mother a sense of community. As Lisa Meeks, a childbirth educator who teaches a popular integrated approach class in the San Francisco Bay Area, put it, "Pregnant women are thirsty for connection with one another. Childbirth instruction, like prenatal exercise classes, is one of the opportunities they have to come together and be there for each other. It's wonderful to see these women be able to confide their fears in each other, reassure each other, or just joke around and release some tension."

In addition, the classes serve a similar function to nesting rituals. Like the search for the perfect stroller, the search for and attendance at a good childbirth class can have a talismanic effect. The act of learning about the progression and terminology of birth offers something to grasp on to when the mind's demons threaten to take over. Though good instruction can't (and shouldn't try) to eliminate all pre-labor anxiety, it can give it constructive focus and manageable scope.

Now, all an expectant mother must do is remember what night of the week she's supposed to show up at her class. And, for that matter, where she last parked her car so she can get there on time. But such seemingly minor chores may present challenges in themselves.

Space Cases

Earlier in this book, it was mentioned that pregnant women, while seeming to develop their intuitive ways of knowing during the course of pregnancy, make a mental trade-off of sorts, becoming to one degree or another more absentminded than before. Though this is one of those phenomena from which many women in pregnancy's earliest stages believe they will somehow be exempt, I have rarely encountered anyone who did not admit that it caught up with her by her eighth month. Indeed even those who generally boast the keenest heads for details, dates, directions, and the like are apt, as pregnancy moves toward its final weeks, to misplace, forget, omit, and confuse things, at least on occasion.

Science corroborates anecdotal evidence here, with controlled testing of cognitive function in pregnant and nonpregnant groups of women showing an increase in the number of errors made by those who were carrying a child.[3] But it's anecdotes which convey the sort of whimsical glitches in which the pregnant mind is likely to engage. For example:

"About six weeks before my delivery date," said 27-year-old Liz, "I was scheduled to attend an orientation at my hospital. I even made my husband reschedule a business trip so we could go together. The night of the orientation, my husband and I were late because when we left the house I forgot some critical forms, pre-certification from my insurance company, on the kitchen table and we had to return to get them. We raced on to the meeting, losing more time when we were stopped on the road for speeding—my husband managed to talk his way out of a ticket by pointing to me and saying, 'We're on our way to the hospital!'—but when we arrived I discovered we were actually a week early. The meeting was the following Thursday. I'd misremembered the date."

"I was shopping for my baby's layette in a department store," recalled 35-year-old Juliette, "and after paying for some items I walked off leaving my purse at the register. The saleswoman tracked me down and gave it back to me, for which I was very grateful. I took the purse, but walked off leaving my packages. Later the same saleswoman found me again. 'Dear,' she said, 'I think you should go home and put your feet up.' Then she asked quite earnestly, 'You do remember where you live, don't you?' "

What exactly causes pregnancy absentmindedness is the subject of endless conversations among pregnant women in the third trimester, who may or may not be amused by their own forgetfulness. One acquaintance of mine offered a rationale which, though obviously tongue-in-cheek, had a nice symmetry. She believed that toward the end of gestation, when the baby has a big spurt of brain growth, the mother's brain power decreases proportionally. Who knows? Perhaps there's only a finite amount of gray matter in the universe, and this is how it gets spread around.

On a more serious note, several women mentioned they had heard that late pregnancy absentmindedness was hormonally caused. Indeed, there seems little doubt among medical professionals that hormonal factors do contribute to or reinforce the phenomenon. (Blame those fluctuating estrogen levels again.)

In addition, it wouldn't do to overlook the level of sleep deprivation common to many pregnant women by the middle of their third trimester. Insufficient sleep is a well-known foe of cognitive function, and it's not surprising many women notice their forgetfulness increase as their babies practice more and more gymnastics at night.

But once again it's doubtful that physiological factors tell the whole story. From a psychological perspective, we might keep in mind Freud's theory of forgetfulness, mix-ups, and "slips." He believed they were often communications from the unconscious, and thought it important to consider the *meaning* of the symptoms evidenced. When a woman forgets the hospital forms necessary to deliver her baby, perhaps it bespeaks some ambivalence about the place she's chosen for delivery, or trepidation about the birth itself. When she forgets her purse and her purchases, perhaps it means she feels not quite ready to tackle the vast responsibilities of motherhood, from the financial overview to the countless daily duties of baby-tending.

Lastly, let's consider absentmindedness from a more ethereal perspective. What if the diminishment of an expectant mother's linear skills is yet another way of her being in sync with her baby? Sure, she might lose track of things, even lose track of time. That's unnerving because for us much of life is spent keeping track of our things and our time. But for the womb's passenger, existence is all about being whole unto oneself. The in vivo infant is without possessions and is free of time's boundaries. Soon the newborn will shoot forth into linearity, growing up, growing older, coming to distinguish between yesterday, today, and tomorrow. But for now the baby, and to some extent the baby's mother, are travelers in the realm of eternity—a realm where keeping track of car keys, credit cards, and Fil-o-Faxes is wholly irrelevant.

Maybe a pregnant woman's absentmindedness is meant to remind her that there is more to life, and certainly more to motherhood, than mastering myriad daily tasks. Perhaps it is meant, literally, to *absent* her constantly chattering *mind* from her soul, to slow her down, and to rehearse her for the months not too far in the future when she will take a respite from the world and bond with her newborn.

Perhaps it is meant to tell her that despite the brain's desire to continue to race, and despite the deadlines that loom, the spirit wants to float a bit. And that even now—especially now—she must remember to take special care of herself.

❖ AN EXPECTANT MOTHER'S PRIVILEGES
   AND PREROGATIVES

When nesting, remember, Mama (yes, that's you) knows best. Many people will offer you suggestions as to what to equip yourself with for baby's homecoming. Sometimes those suggestions will feel right to you, but sometimes they won't. Once again, follow your instincts. Buy only what fits *your* taste, lifestyle, and budget. Don't overspend on status symbols for their own sake, and don't feel pressured into buying trendy items because of self-righteous sermons. Babies don't know or care a whit about price tags, status, or political correctness. (Happily so, for their innocence is their most winning feature.)

Finally, keep in mind you can't anticipate all your infant's needs in advance. Relax. The stores will still be open after you bring your baby home. (And rest assured that you will be deluged with mail-order catalogues to boot.)

Get informed about breast-feeding from as many sources as possible. When our mothers had us, breast-feeding was definitely "out." Now it's definitely "in." Its well-publicized health benefits are frequently cited by pediatricians and midwives. And even baby formula manufacturers tell us "breast milk is best." It's nice that Mother Nature's beverage of choice is finally getting the respect it deserves. Nonetheless a word must be said as a caution to anyone who feels they "should" nurse their baby purely because of social pressure. The word is *don't*. That is, don't breast-feed because of what others think.

Breast-feeding is an enormous commitment on every level. Is it worth it? Yes, if you have time, patience, and ability to tolerate frustration in the early weeks (before your milk supply stabilizes and before you are able to distinguish between your baby's various cues).

Get as much knowledge as you can ahead of time. Talk to as many nursing mothers as possible about what's really involved, and consult books which will help you visualize whether nursing will fit into your life. (See Suggestions for Further Reading in the back of this book for sources.) If you want to give it a go, fine. However, if after all your research, you believe you would otherwise make a much more agreeable parent by having a bottle-fed baby (who Dad could also feed and who would in all likelihood sleep for somewhat longer intervals as a result of feeling more full), do what you think will serve you and your family best.

And if you can't decide just yet, consider leaving the decision-making door open. Since you won't really know how, or if, nursing will work for you and your baby until you attempt it, you may want to start out breast-feeding, knowing you can change your mind later. (The same can't be said of bottle-feeding.) But in any case, remember that there is a choice here and it is yours.

It's your baby shower—say what you need. If your friends and relations are going to celebrate your impending motherhood with a gift-giving party, don't be afraid to make your needs known. If you already have tons of hand-me-down baby clothes, spread the word so you're not inundated with more tiny T-shirts than you'll ever need. If you are really in need of one big-ticket item, suggest (or ask the shower host to suggest) that people chip in or contribute what they can toward a gift certificate.

And here's a fresh idea that seems well worth considering. Heidi Beigel, head of the California-based Fourth Trimester company, one of many new organizations which are springing up to assist new mothers, suggests getting shower guests to give vouchers for personal services, collectible "on demand" after the baby is born. At her own shower, for example, "one friend volunteered to bring over a meal once a week for six weeks, one offered to do the laundry, one offered to sit with the baby while I napped."

As long as you're shopping, buy yourself a teddy bear too. Baby isn't the only one who needs something to hold on to. During the last trimester, you'll appreciate "comfort objects" of your own. The suggestion of buying a "teddy bear" for yourself can be taken literally or metaphorically. It can mean gifting yourself with a good novel to keep you company as you wait for the baby's arrival. It can mean getting a comfy robe for the hospital, or a pretty, loose-fitting outfit so you can come home feeling somewhat put together. In any case, don't neglect your current wants and needs while trying to guess what the baby's will be. The best thing for baby to come home to is a mother who is not already fatigued and overwrought from running around trying to make everything "perfect."

Choose a childbirth class that neither fills you with fear nor attempts to rid you of it. When interviewing instructors for prepared childbirth it's important to find one who you feel you can trust, and whose approach in not off-putting to you based on your own priorities and sensibilities. But beware anyone who tries to take all your fear away, or who makes you feel silly for having it in the first place. As Gayle Peterson writes in her book, *Birthing Normally,* when it comes to having a baby: "A complete absence of fear is as worrisome as total fear."[4] One should approach birthing with an appropriate amount of awe for the powerful, fundamentally unpredictable process that is about to take place. To assume it is totally under one's control is really to be *un*prepared.

Enjoy your nonlinearity. Okay, so you misplaced your address book for the fifth time and forgot to check the oil in your car. The world won't stop spinning if you wait to make a few phone calls (that book will turn up sooner or later!), and throw yourself on the mercy of your local gas station attendants. Sure, you can beat up on yourself for letting some of life's endless chores slip through the cracks. Or you can take a breather and log some quality daydream time. Consider the latter course and go, as they say, with the flow.

It's natural to feel mildly compulsive in the home stretch, natural to feel like hunting down the perfect cradle, stalking the snuggest snowsuit, natural to want to get familiarized with the mechanics and the vocabulary of birthing. But it's also natural to feel a little bit as if complete control of your life eludes you, as if your energy—revitalized though it may be—is somewhat scattered, and as if you are "not quite yourself." You're not. You are yourself and your baby. Your child's energy is growing stronger and stronger now. And he or she too has a deadline to meet. . . .

9 Born at the Right Time

I could hear time, a machine sound, I could feel creation, myself in place for the first time.

—SHARON DOUBIAGO
South America Mi Hija

When I first became pregnant I knew virtually nothing about the birth process, except that it seemed mysterious and frightening. But by the ninth month of my pregnancy, I had gathered as much knowledge as I could. Now I had a clear idea of how I wanted my birth to go.

In my imagination it went just so: An onset of contractions a week or so before my due date (because I tend to be impatient by nature and assumed my child would be the same). A predictable succession of increasingly frequent contractions taking me to six centimeters dilation while still laboring at home, doing relaxation exercises. A quick trip to my hospital's lovely and quiet Alternative Birthing Center, where the admittance nurse and my midwife would nod approvingly at my progress and my husband would comment on what a trooper I'd been.

Next: A challenging but manageable (and totally drug-free) journey into and out of the transition phase. An hour or so of strenuous pushing (through which I maintained my "trooper" status). A perfect baby put immediately to my breast and left to nestle contentedly in my arms without being swooped off to the nursery that awaited infants born in the hospital's more conventional Labor and Delivery wing.

Wrong.

In reality, my labor went like so: A tentative onset of contractions some ten days after my due date was past. An erratic progression of contractions growing closer together, then further apart for over twenty-four confusing hours. A trip to the hospital where it was confirmed I was only one centimeter dilated. A mild sedative to try to determine if this flukey labor was false, and, if so, to make it subside. A trip back home to undergo another night of oddly spaced labor pains and a slow leak in my amniotic fluid. A readmission to the hospital the next afternoon for an IV drip of pitocin because I'd agreed (and who wouldn't, by now?) it was in the best interests of all to jump-start this rambling labor. Then, a room in the conventional Labor and Delivery wing because the Alternative Birthing Center was reserved for the chemical-free.

Next, a ride on the medical merry-go-round: A pain reliever, because the pitocin made the contractions abnormally intense. A three-hour-plus spell of pushing. A final tug with forceps, because my baby—perfect though he did turn out to be—decided to cock his head in the birth canal to have a final look around. And, at last, a brief chance to ogle and snuggle my adorable new son before he was whisked off to the nursery after all.

My baby was whole and healthy—and cuter than a tree full of koala bears—all of which made me glad beyond words. But at the same time I felt mad, and sad, and even a little guilty. Sad because my birth had been "medicalized," which I had expressly attempted to avoid, but, due to unusual circumstances, couldn't seem to. Mad because those same circumstances meant I hadn't gotten to use the ABC and therefore had to meet and greet my baby only briefly, according to the very different high-tech protocol in Labor and Delivery. Guilty because I felt I had somehow let myself and my husband and our baby down by not having proceeded according to plan. For days, weeks, I questioned why things went as they did. I postulated theories.

I surmised that my labor was so strangely drawn-out partly because when I'd first called my midwife to tell her it had begun I discovered she had had to go out of town and would not be back until the following evening. Although her colleague, a female obstetrician I respected, was on duty, I was bereft. I wanted my midwife, to whom I'd felt so close. I needed her! I wished so hard for her presence that perhaps my body stalled for time in order to make it so.

I thought too that to some extent my own unresolved uncertainties about my ability to be a good mother—actually a great mother, for deep down I'd hoped to be nothing less— played a role in delaying my child's birth. No matter how much I'd attempted to healthily acknowledge and process my anxieties for the nine months preceding my son's arrival, part of me wanted, at the last minute, more time still. (Greatness, after all, is an elusive goal. And I now know that if my son had waited for me to achieve anything approximating it, he'd be waiting still.)

But what about my son, and his own role in this birthing saga? After all, it was his drama as much as my own. I thought he'd come early, and move along speedily. But he had his own ideas. (Still does!) That's part of what I'd neglected to consider. If indeed, as I like to think, each child has his or her own karmic purpose, his or her special destiny to fulfill, that destiny must begin to unfold at birth. Perhaps my baby knew, deep in his soul, when it was exactly the "right" time to emerge from the womb. From his perspective, he was born not a moment too late, nor a moment too soon.

All of these seemed to me like sound reasons why my labor unfolded the way it did. Even today, after much time spent mulling it all over, I do not discount any of them, and believe they all played a part. But the more time elapses, the more I am also convinced that each childbirth, like the months of pregnancy before it, occurs in a particular way to impart valuable lessons that need to be learned. One of the things my child's birth taught me was humility.

Before the birth I sat in my ego, in my willful mind, and wrote out my birth plan, describing, essentially, how the life force would manifest itself in me and how I, and those around me, would respond. That force, however, is so potent and so purposeful that any attempt to script it indelibly in ink is a setup for disappointment.

It is one thing to be informed and educated about birth. (I have never regretted being so for a moment, for it enabled me to be clear about my preferences and to take an active role in making certain choices, even when my range of options grew narrower than I might have hoped.) But it is another thing to be so wed to an image of what constitutes an ideal birth that anything else registers as a defeat.

If I had to do over again, or if I have another child, I would not have a birth "plan" so much as a birth "wish." I would hope to remember that no matter how much one knows, and ought to know, every birth is a doorway to the unknown. And I would do my best to bear in mind that all births are deep learning experiences for those who choose to be open to them.

Looked at from this point of view, my child's birth was a perfect birth. For it was just what it needed to be to teach his mother a thing or two. . . .

Women on the Verge

From the first prenatal checkup, a mother-to-be is given a "due date." Forty weeks are counted from the first day of her last menstrual period before conception, and she is told that at the end of that time, more or less, her baby will arrive. Everyone is aware that the calculation of due dates is hardly a precision science, and most everyone has heard their share of cultural and family lore to assist them in making their own predictions about their babies' birthdays (for instance, "Babies come with the full moon," or "First babies are always late," or "We Jones women are always three weeks early."). But in any case, it is typical to enter one's ninth month of pregnancy with at least a vague target time frame in mind for the big event. Bags are packed, layettes are laundered, and, in an information-age development, husbands are equipped with beepers so they can be contacted anywhere, at any time.

Some women, even if they've remained highly active throughout their pregnancies, choose to hand off some of their many nonmaternal responsibilities to others as their due dates approach. Others forge ahead full steam—or try to—determined not to disrupt their routines any more than is absolutely necessary. But no matter what chores and habits one chooses to continue or discontinue, some emotional disruption is inevitable. It's not uncommon for a particular kind of ambivalence to manifest itself in the eleventh hour, and for a woman to simultaneously long for both a speeding up and a slowing down of the final phase of the pregnancy process.

On the one hand, she wants to get it over with. She is anxious to put the physical cumbersomeness of late pregnancy behind her. She is extremely eager and curious to meet her child at long last. And if she has already taken a leave from her job, she may feel bored and restless, pining for her new duties to begin.

If she goes past her due date (meaning her "official" one or the one she informally has targeted in her mind) she may well become especially impatient. Anyone who has spent time in the waiting room of an obstetrical office knows that glum *enough already* expression that past-due women tend to sport. A past-due mother-to-be may be soliciting all kinds of folkloric advice as to how to "shake things up in there" and try everything from herbal concoctions to bumpy car rides to particular foods which are rumored to do the trick. (An L.A. restaurant called Caioti got its fifteen minutes of fame in 1993 when *Newsweek* reported that enceinte women were flocking to sample its romaine and watercress salad with balsamic vinegar dressing—complete with "secret" ingredient— because they believed it instigated contractions.)[1]

Even the most impatient, most overripe mother-to-be, however, may harbor sentiments antithetical to those which exhort her baby to move this business along. An expectant woman, at the very last, may on some level wish that her pregnancy could go on forever. She has grown used to having a baby inside her, but may not feel ready to take care of its many needs once it is physically separate from her. She has a set way of doing things, a set way of relating to her spouse (and to her other children if she is already a mother), and she can't help but feel somewhat reluctant to step out of these well-worn grooves. Perhaps she has gotten lots of positive attention during her pregnancy and she is likely aware that she is about to be nudged from center stage. And of course, she will now have to contend with labor and childbirth, which is few people's idea of a balmy day at the beach.

Naturally no pregnancy will go on forever. No matter how many complex and conflicting emotions a woman is feeling, sooner or later her baby's birthday will arrive. And unless she has, for medical reasons, arranged ahead of time for the induction of labor or the scheduling of a cesarian, there is simply no way to preordain precisely when that will be. Nor is there really any way to know how labor will go, and how a woman will respond to the many things that may happen during its course.

The Unfolding

Livingston Jones, an observer among the Tlinget tribe of Alaska in the early part of this century, wrote in his study of that people: "The vast majority of Tlinget women suffer very little and some not at all, when their children are born. They have been known to give birth sleeping."[2] One gets the distinct impression that Jones never actually saw a Tlinget woman give birth in her sleep, and that this tale is an embellished legend meant to convey a Tlinget cultural imperative. (Remember, tribal peoples often treated childbirth as an opportunity for women to display culturally sanctioned acts of courage, such as refraining from crying out during labor.) It is, of course, wonderful to imagine rolling over, having a snore and a stretch and . . . a baby. Wonderful, but hardly realistic.

Challenging, effortful childbirth is, as the anthropologist and physician Melvin Konner has put it, "a legacy of human evolution." The human pelvis had to become adapted for weight-bearing when Homo sapiens began to walk upright. Its new shorter, stockier shape made it less than ideal for birthgiving, and resulted in what's known as the cephalopelvic "crunch" of birth. Meanwhile, our species was evolving larger heads to accommodate larger brains. Add the two developments together and you get, as Konner says, an "evolutionary squeeze."[3]

Certainly our mythical Tlinget woman may have begun her labor in her sleep, just as many women in our society do. For labor often begins when a woman is relaxed. But even if she is sleeping soundly as a stone, she won't remain that way for long.

Whenever labor starts it is because a complex interaction of mother's and baby's hormones have started a ball rolling. Momentum builds, and over the next hours, be they a great many or comparatively few, the baby progresses through a series of postural changes—engagement, descent, flexion, internal rotation, external rotation, extension, expulsion. (The catchy medical school mnemonic for this: Every Damn Fool in Egypt Eats Eggs.)[4]

For her part, the mother will respond strongly not only with her body but with her emotions. Such is the way humans respond to any stress, and birth is a natural stress.

The laboring woman will gradually move from a stance of nervous excitement (perhaps even tinged with elation, because *hey, this is finally, actually happening*) to intense seriousness. She will cease going about other activities between contractions, she will concentrate avidly, and grunt or moan loudly. She will, without question, lose her sense of humor. In fact, if she still finds much of anything amusing, she's likely got quite a ways to go.

> "I remember," said 33-year-old Dorothy, "thinking I was far along in labor—and thinking hey, this isn't so bad—when my husband pulled out his Polaroid and I started mugging for the camera. My obstetrician saw this, turned to my husband, and said, 'Oh, oh. She's still smiling. It's going to be a long night.' "

She will very often snap at her husband, even if such outbursts are out of character for her.

"My wife never uses four-letter words under normal circumstances," said 37-year-old Jeremiah, father of four daughters. "If
she says, 'Oh shoot,' you know she's really upset. But when she's
in labor she curses like a trooper, usually at me because 'it's all my
fault.' The first time, I took offense. Now I know it's part of the
deal, and it makes me think, 'Oh, good, the baby's coming soon.' "

At a certain point, she will probably begin to lose faith in
her ability to get this job done. She may feel like she simply can't
summon up any more effort. But as childbirth educator Susan
McCutcheon-Rosegg has pointed out, this phase of self-doubt is
often, paradoxically, yet another emotional signpost of progress.[5] It is often when a woman thinks she just can't take it anymore that she is on the threshold of pushing her baby out.

"It felt like I had been pushing forever," recalled Rosalind, who
gave birth to her first child at 39. "I remember saying to my midwife, 'I can't do it. I just can't do it.' She looked at me and said,
'Ros, who else is going to do it?' About two minutes later, my baby
was born."

Amazing as it may seem while one is in the tumultuous midst
of labor, sooner or later, one way or another, out the baby will
come. Mother and child will at long last officially meet. And
although, in a certain sense, they have been long and intimately
acquainted, what a moment this is! Many women are moved in
ways they never imagined possible before. They are moved beyond words, past tears, into something wondrous and inexpress-
ible. For they have had a hand in the making of a miracle. They
have come out the other side of an event which was both a sacra-
ment and an ordeal. And, despite their deepest doubts and fears,
they have lived to tell.

Later, with the drama of birth in its denouement, friends and
relations will eagerly call for news. They wish to know baby's
gender, name, and birth weight. They want to know that everything and everyone's okay. And some will also want a brief
"recap" from mother about the details of her baby's birth. "So,"
they'll ask, "how was the delivery?"

Many a new mother has commented what an odd word *de-*

livery is to describe the childbirth process. It conjures up images of speed and ease. *Ta da!* A wriggling bundle is picked up in the cabbage patch and dropped off by the stork, or perhaps even by Federal Express. But of course that's not anything like what has just occurred. What occurred, as far as the new mother is concerned, was more along the lines of a personal odyssey than an efficiently accomplished errand.

How she will recall and recount this odyssey, from her first contraction to the moment when she held her baby in her arms, depends on many variables. Very often, a woman enters into the process of childbirth with expectations of how events will unfold. Each stage of the birth can be a point of coincidence between expectations and reality, or it can be a point of divergence. And how a woman feels about her labor forever after can depend on just how much of each there is.

Points of Divergence

Expectations and actuality tend to coincide when a woman who wants a high-tech birth gets one and feels it served her well, or when a woman who wants a natural birth accomplishes her goal without undue medical intervention. In fact, the conclusion of Robbie E. Davis-Floyd, the cultural anthropologist who chronicled women's reactions to childbirth in her book *Birth as an American Rite of Passage*, was that "the single factor that most influences the conceptual outcome of a woman's birth is the correspondence between the technocratic model of reality dominant in the hospital and the belief system she herself holds when she enters the hospital."[6]

When hopes and outcome are in harmony, childbirth tends to be experienced and recalled as a nontraumatic event. While it may be remembered as intense, even extremely difficult, its overall emotional effect is benign. But when a woman counts on one sort of birth and gets another, the divergence can take a heavy emotional toll.

Divergence between expectation and reality in childbirth can have many causes. In some instances, it occurs because of a lack of consensus between a woman and her caregivers once she has entered the environment where she has elected to give birth. Like Davis-Floyd, I encountered a number of women who were unhappy with their childbirth experiences because they perceived the system as having failed them. For some women I spoke with, this was because they felt entitled to, and believed they would get, complete and swift relief from pain. They were dissatisfied with relief they felt came too late or that left them with so-called "hot spots" of sensitivity.

"My doctor said I could have an epidural anytime I wanted," recalled 29-year-old Meredith. "But when I said I wanted one *right now* they couldn't find the anesthesiologist. By the time he turned up, it hardly made any difference. I don't know if it was because it was so late in the game or what, but part of me felt numb and part of me didn't at all. Plus now everything slowed way down because it was harder for me to push. Why didn't anyone tell me this sort of things wasn't foolproof?"

In most instances, however, dissatisfaction with the system was felt by women who wanted, and anticipated, a far more intervention-free experience than they actually got. Sometimes divergences arose when a practitioner a woman had counted on, and come to certain understandings with, was ultimately unavailable:

"I told my doctor explicitly," recalled 33-year-old Candice, "that I wanted to try to avoid being hooked up to IV's and fetal monitors and such. I wanted to be able to birth in a position other than the 'lying on your back' position that has become routine in hospitals, since I believed strongly that lying down lengthened and potentially complicated labor. My doctor agreed I could do the birth 'my way' so long as there were no complications. But as it turned out, I got to the hospital way ahead of my doctor, who was tending to an emergency. By the time he arrived, his backup had insisted on hooking me up to all the machines I wanted to avoid—not because there were complications but because, he'd explained, this was standard operating procedure in this hospital and he wasn't aware of my doctor's agreement to depart from it. He basically said, this is the way we do it here and there's no use arguing. So I gave birth feeling like part of a machine, and feeling totally manipulated."

Sometimes a practitioner, once at the hospital, seemed to subscribe to a different philosophy than the one espoused at the woman's prenatal visits:

"One of the things I really wanted to avoid was an episiotomy," said 28-year-old Jamie. "The very thought terrified me. I had told my doctor this early on and she had said, 'Well, I only do them when absolutely necessary.' But when it came time to push the baby out, she said matter-of-factly, 'Well, now we'll do a little episiotomy.' I reminded her she said *only if it was absolutely necessary*, but she said it was, in her opinion. My baby was just over six and a half pounds. Since then, I've met women who had babies bigger than mine and who gave birth without episiotomies.

"I had spent months doing squatting exercises and perineal massage. I still think I could have been spared the episiotomy. But I found out later that my doctor performed this procedure on nearly all her patients. I think she hadn't really taken me seriously!"

Was I to Blame?

Not all women whose birth experiences did not meet their espectations blame the system, or blame it entirely. Some blame themselves, and experience remorse at their "failure" to birth their child in a particular manner.

"I made a big deal out of not wanting to use any sort of drugs during childbirth," said 27-year-old Michele. "But by the time I was six centimeters I was begging for an epidural. Later, I felt like I wimped out. I'm sure it was all because I wasn't able to relax properly. I must admit I've always tended to carry any mental tension in my body—I get backaches when I'm stressed, for example. But I thought of childbirth as a good opportunity to break this pattern. I really practiced labor breathing techniques diligently, and I thought I could handle it. I couldn't. It was a blow."

"After I had my cesarian," said 31-year-old Beverly, "I felt like my body had betrayed me. I dilated fully but then I just couldn't push the baby out. I think it was my own fear that got me stuck. Part of me was really scared, I think, because a neighbor of mine had talked to me a lot during my pregnancy about how excruciating *she* found the pushing stage of labor. I wish I'd done something except let her talk on while I suffered in silence, but I never mentioned my feelings to her or anyone else. Anyway, my surgery went alright, but it left me so weak I couldn't really take care of my new daughter the way I wanted to for the first week or two of her life. I felt so impotent. I wish I hadn't let my dread get the better of me."

The reactions of these two women illustrate how a woman's self-esteem may be impacted by the choices she makes during the course of her labor. To not live up to one's expectations of oneself during childbirth can potentially have long-lasting detrimental effects on a new mother's psyche, causing her to question her strength, her resolve, and even her capability for parenting.

What a catch-22 a birth mother finds herself in. She may believe that her emotions (perhaps the very emotions she finds unappealing in herself and tries hardest to repress under normal circumstances) undermined her intentions. And, in some ways, she may be right. It is never prudent to discount the complex relationship between mind and body. Certainly an exorbitant degree of anxiety and fear (especially when these emotions have gone largely unacknowledged) can impact the course of labor just as they can impact any other physical process, from the functioning of the immune system to the achievement of sexual satisfaction. But reproaching herself for anything and everything that happened during her baby's birth can make her feel more helpless than ever.

At a certain point—the point where a reasonable acknowledgment that one's emotions were part of a causative chain of events turns to a punitive sense of self-recrimination—one must draw the line. The acknowledgment of the role of one's psyche in childbirth is genuinely useful only to the extent that it results in a new degree of self-understanding which in turn can foster constructive growth.

For example, a woman like Michele, who believes her habit of holding tension in her body undermined her intentions to have a drug-free labor, might resolve to find long-term ways of dealing with such a habit, such as making relaxation and meditation a regular part of her life. A women like Beverly, who feels her fear stymied her resolve, might, for future pregnancies, try harder to discuss her fears ahead of time, to set limits on people whose "terror tales" haunt her, and to keep her empathy for another mother from turning into dire prognostications for herself and her baby.

And a woman like myself, who believes that lingering unrealistic expectations of herself as a mother contributed to drawing out her labor, might resolve as I in fact have to continue addressing and exploring this issue within herself as she raises her child.

Similarly, the act of finding fault with the system, as an end in itself, is likely to leave one feeling victimized and powerless. However, a woman can choose to convert any residual anger into a useful catalyst for change. She may make it a point to inform her practitioner of her grievances (perhaps this will help other expectant mothers in that practitioner's care). And she may resolve to better protect her interests in any future pregnancies by making sure, for example, that she is acquainted and feels comfortable with any potential backup practitioners ahead of time, or that she asks her practitioner more specific questions than she had before (such as "What is your definition of *absolutely necessary?*").

A Matter of Perspective

Along with all of this, however, a woman must bring a realistic perspective to her childbirth. To paraphrase the well-known Serenity Prayer, it is well and good to have the strength to change what one can, but also good to acknowledge that there are some things one simply cannot change. The truth is even if a woman was the most well-informed, self-confident, physically fit, pain-tolerant, relaxation-competent mother-to-be in the world, it is entirely possible she *still* might have a complicated birth. Maybe because her baby decided to do a last-minute somersault. Maybe because of the particular shape of her pelvis. Maybe because the child came unexpectedly early or unexpectedly quickly. Maybe just because.

Nature and birth are unpredictable. Babies are themselves unpredictable. This has always been so. And no matter what techniques we devise for birthgiving, from the most natural and unfettered approach to the most relentlessly high-tech, it will always be so. *But just because things didn't turn out as one expected doesn't mean one has failed.* Quite the opposite. For one has succeeded in having a baby—and in gaining a valuable learning opportunity.

To be sure, during labor thoughts, feelings, and physical sensations seem to blend together in a rising crescendo. A woman is immersed in the intensity of the entire experience, and in its midst—or even in the first few hours after its completion—it would be impossible for her to sort out all the many factors that coincided to make her particular birth evolve the way it did. In retrospect, however, she may well be able to make a certain sense of the events which occurred. And if she finds that her birth experience has left her with sad or angry feelings she cannot shake, she will find it especially valuable to do just that.

By waiting awhile and then reviewing her recollections, and by asking for the input of her husband, her labor coach, and her physician or midwife, she can begin to piece together a narrative—her birth tale—which includes some ideas about various causes and effects. She can allow herself a period of anger and allow herself sadness, for not to honor one's feelings would be counterproductive, but she can then transform those feelings into positive actions.

She can distinguish, at least to some extent, what was inevitable from what might have been preventable. She can take steps to try to work on issues over which she can exert some influence (such as vowing to negotiate the medical system to her greater advantage next time, or to explore further any personal anxieties which she believes may have gotten her "stuck" in labor in one way or another). And she can begin to let the matters which were beyond her sphere of influence go, accepting that some things "just happen" or happen for reasons beyond our comprehension.

Most useful of all, she can ask herself what lessons her birth may possibly have been meant to teach her. Then, rather than rebuking herself, she can begin to incorporate those lessons into her daily life.

For example, 35-year-old Penny believed her birth lesson was "be more assertive." She resolved to try.

> "By agreeing to some of the interventions I did, I think I made things easier for my doctor, rather than for me and my baby. Now I am aware of my tendency to defer to authority and I work hard at not giving in to people because they are powerful figures or 'experts.'"

Thirty-nine-year-old Danielle believed her birth lesson was "be more patient." She's working at it.

> "I insisted on going to the hospital with the first contraction. They sent me home. Two hours later I went back. They sent me home again. The third time, they took me in, though it was still way too soon. I could have been in my own cozy living room, or in a nice warm shower. Instead I was in the hospital for what seemed like forever, and I think the environment there just made me more nervous, which ultimately worked against me and dragged my labor out. Now I have a baby and I see how important patience is. Babies do things in their own time. I can't make my daughter cut her teeth any faster or take solid food before she's ready. If I try, I'll make us both unhappy. It's a struggle, but I now see that the right time for things makes itself known."

Lydia, who gave birth for the first time at 28 years of age, felt, as she put it, "more proud to be a woman, and more connected to other women all over the world." Her lesson was about both self-worth and community. But on a more specific level, she felt childbirth enabled her "to reconnect" with one woman in particular.

"My mother and I, though not entirely estranged, had a superficial relationship for many years until I had my baby," she said. "I held a lot of things against her. It wasn't like my giving birth made everything okay between us, but it did inspire me to try and deepen our relationship. I realized that, no matter what else had happened, she had done this incredible thing for me. I could picture her as scared and overwhelmed as I was as a new mother, and I suddenly wanted to let her know she hadn't done it all in vain, that we could share something."

The lessons cited are specific to individual circumstances, but their collective purpose is the same. They are prescriptions for healing the past and facing the future.

By *processing* the emotional realities of her baby's birth, as these women did, rather than suppressing them or simply replaying any disappointments Ancient Mariner style, a new mother will be better equipped to face the new challenges which lie before her.

For make no mistake, plenty of them remain.

Aftermath

On the road to womanhood, most of us have, at one point or another, been exposed to *Good Earth* type stories of hearty peasant women who had a baby one minute and returned to plowing a field the next. We've also heard family lore of great-great-grandmothers who gave birth, jumped up, turned over the turkey, and scrubbed the kitchen floor. While we may not wish that all the details of such amazing scenarios would be applicable to us (given a choice, we'd leave the plowing until later, thank you), most everyone would like to bounce back from labor with alacrity.

But as in childbirth, wishes and reality may not always be congruent. It's true that just after giving birth, a woman may well experience a brief high. Typically, she is relieved that her difficult task has been completed, and thrilled to bits that the product of her labor has all its sweet little fingers and precious little toes and Daddy's big dimple and Great-grandma's nose. But soon enough her joy may be tempered with other feelings.

For one thing, she is physically drained. Even the most optimum of labors is an exhausting enterprise. In addition, her hormonal state is experiencing a rapid and massive shift. Within twenty-four hours after delivery estrogen and progesterone levels, which were at their peak in late pregnancy, have dropped dramatically (both because the glands are producing far less and because the placenta is gone). This chemical alteration is considered by many the prime cause of the so-called "baby blues," the emotional dip which commonly occurs between the second and fifth postpartum day and which is estimated to affect 80 to 90 percent of new mothers.[7] (Baby blues are technically not the same as more severe postpartum depression, which the next chapter will address.)

But once again, physiology doesn't tell the whole story. The immediately postpartum mother has psychological and social reasons for the blues as well. She has just endured an event of marathon proportions. Unlike the marathon runner, however, she has not been cheered by vast crowds, taken out for brunch, and sent home for some well-deserved R&R. Instead she has been bumped from star status to a supporting role, and been fêted with a tray of hospital food. As for rest and recreation, it's not likely she'll have much chance for either, as throngs of well-wishers drop by to coo at her newborn and as hospital staffers, for reasons best known to themselves, do their usual 4 A.M. blood-pressure checks.

In addition, a woman fresh out of the childbirth experience may feel alienated from her body. Granted it's been the vehicle for a heaven-sent blessing, but, hey, isn't it supposed to return to normal already? Instead, the recently delivered woman finds her body, contrary to her deepest hopes, has not sprung back instantly into pre-pregnancy condition but rather is languishing in an odd state of semi-deflation.

Will things ever return to the way they were before? she wonders. (And realizes, with a start, that it's almost impossible to remember exactly *what* she was like before.) Will her husband ever find her sexually attractive again? (Sure, he's looking at her with that adoring light in his eyes, but is that because she's a *mother,* rather than a lover?) And, while she's on the subject, just whose breasts are these, anyhow? (They're engorged beyond anything she's ever imagined and she instantly knows that the nursing bras she ordered will be several sizes too small.) And what on earth is she supposed to do about a wardrobe? (As one woman said, "I just can't bring myself to face wearing the same clothes on the way 'down' that I wore on the way 'up.'")

Last but without a doubt not least, a new mother's "blues" can be influenced by the emotionally overwhelming fact that she is now—all at once—so profoundly responsible for someone so helpless, so unimaginably tiny and completely dependent. Fatigued though she may be, the mother must quickly begin to accommodate her baby's seemingly limitless demands. She must accept that carrying this baby for nine months and then giving birth to it was only the beginning of a lifelong commitment. (As a friend of mine who gave birth late one Friday night put it, "When Monday rolled around I kept thinking, this wasn't just something I did over the weekend, this was eternal.")

Having a baby is more than a weekend jaunt, indeed. It is a radical undertaking. And the new mother must come to terms with the fact that even when her dazed and dozing tiny infant becomes a boisterous toddler, a savvy schoolchild, an annoying adolescent, and a full-fledged grown-up she will always be a mother, albeit not so "new" anymore.

As a mother, your duties will be innumerable. And you must take each and every one of them to heart. But at no time, particularly not at this very early, very critical stage, must you obliterate yourself in the process. For the best gift you can give your baby is your own self-respect. So as you head home with your baby and begin one of the most significant phases of both your lives, you can best rise to the occasion not by dismissing your needs, but by dignifying them, and by remembering to love yourself as you love your child. For in many regards, though you are now no longer physically joined, you are still inextricably merged.

❖ A NEW MOTHER'S PRIVILEGES AND PREROGATIVES

Allow for the unplanned in your birth plan. As you head toward the final weeks of your pregnancy, you may be encouraged by your childbirth educator or practitioner to draft a birth plan, documenting for the record your preferences for labor and delivery. This is a good way of making sure everyone involved is aware of what you'd prefer. But remember that what one prefers is not always what occurs. Maybe your wishes will mesh totally with reality, which would be wonderful. But maybe Mother Nature will throw you a curve. Or maybe your baby will have a different agenda than you. Or maybe your baby will change your mind midway through labor about what it is you want after all. John Lennon once said, "Life is what happens while you're making other plans." Many mothers could tell you that birth, too, often happens while you're making other plans.

Work at processing your birth once it's over. Every new mother deserves an opportunity to get a handle on what happened during the birth of her baby and, to the extent that it's possible to know, on why things happened as they did. Whether you feel a sense of triumph or pain, or some combination of both, you owe it to yourself to come to terms with whatever happened so you can learn from it, put it aside, and move on. If no one offers you such an opportunity (and they may not, for our society is strangely better at allowing people to access their feelings after a death than after a birth), create opportunities for yourself. Talk things over with your husband and perhaps others to whom you feel close. Meet with your childbirth practitioner for a "debriefing," and get answers to any lingering questions you have about what took place. Call up your childbirth educator and discuss your experience.

If the idea appeals to you, consider sharing your birth tale with other new mothers in a group setting arranged for that purpose (perhaps a childbirth educator or labor coach can help arrange this).

Remember, every woman who has given birth, whether under largely positive circumstances or difficult ones, wants to tell her story. Doing so in a caring, emotionally safe situation where one is free to feel one's feelings is a good way to keep from holding on to emotional residue indefinitely.

Absorb the lessons of your labor, whatever they may be. Annie Fox, a New York-based prenatal counselor and labor coach, told me, "Everyone dies during childbirth." She was speaking metaphorically, of course, and meant that in a certain sense, one's old self is replaced by a new self. Like all transformative experiences, labor is rich with meaning. And like all such experiences, there is simply no question of "failure."

Ask yourself what your child's birth may have been meant to show you. If you pose this question with a sincere intent to gain knowledge, the answers will likely come clear after a time.

What you learn is yours to keep and savor. It is one of the gifts the universe gives you when you give birth to a baby. The other gift is the baby itself. With these gifts to cherish, how can one possibly have failed?

Don't expect a second miracle from your body—at least not right away. Your body has just spent nine months growing a baby. Now it has sent that baby forth into the world. It has done an unbelievably amazing job. But now it needs to rest, and to take its own good time getting back to the way it was before.

No, you can't get into your pre-pregnancy jeans, let alone your pre-pregnancy bras, before you leave the hospital (and maybe not for months afterwards).

No, you can't do your sit-ups yet. Maybe even walking won't be your idea of a good time for the next week or so.

And yes, you're going to feel weary, and you'll probably experience some side effects from your latest jaunt on the hormonal roller coaster.

Just do your best to give your body the sustenance it needs and allow it to readjust in a natural fashion. Don't be intimidated by stories of so-and-so's friend's cousin who allegedly taught aerobics and modeled swimsuits on her fifth postpartum day, any more than you would be by those tall tales of ancestors who sprang from the labor bed to hoe potatoes. You ought not consider yourself a participant in any "bouncing back" competition here, either with ghosts of the past or peers of the present. Just as each woman's womb grows a unique baby, each woman's body must heal and restore itself in its own way.

Welcome your baby well. If you had your baby in a conventional setting you were likely not offered any meaningful postpartum rituals, except for being given a few iron pills and a soft cushion to sit on. Your baby probably wasn't welcomed with a meaningful ritual either, except for being rated with an Apgar score. But you and your spouse (and your other children if you already have any) can devise your own rituals and foster your own private traditions. Think about ways in which you can make events like naming your child, introducing her to her siblings, or bringing her home from the hospital, a memorable time. If there were parts of the labor and delivery experience you found disappointing, see if you can compensate for some of them now, for example, by bringing your baby home to dimmed lights and soft music that it might have been nice to have had at the birth, or by simply allowing a few days for you and your baby to do little else except snuggle together.

If you found the spiritual aspect of your birth hard to get in touch with in all the medical hullabaloo, and if that aspect is important to you, allow time after the birth to give thanks in a way that is appropriate for you, and to welcome your baby in your family's spiritual tradition. If you don't have a spiritual tradition, but have (perhaps as a direct result of carrying and bearing your child) become interested in pursuing one, this could be a good time to begin thinking about ways in which you might incorporate this dimension into your lives.

This is your baby's inauguration into your family, and your inauguration as this baby's mother. Make it special, but keep things simple and comfortable. You don't need a lot of fanfare to mark this occasion, but you do need to ackowledge the significance of all that has happened, and all that still awaits you.

Don't underestimate the depth of the ongoing changes of which you are in the midst. The next few months are sure to test you, and you will need to draw strength from as many sources as possible.

10 Sleepless Dreams

> Motherhood is a storm, a seizure: It is like weather.
> Nights of high wind, followed by calm mornings of
> brilliant sunshine that gives way to tropical rain, or
> blinding snow.
>
> —LAURIE COLWIN
> *A Big Storm Knocked It Over*

*A*t 2:00 or 3:00 or 4:00 A.M. *(I can't remember which, and
it no longer mattered anyhow) my six-week-old son, Skyler,
woke me with a piecing cry straight to the left eardrum. He'd
fallen asleep on my pillow after the last feeding, and I had
fallen into something sort of resembling sleep. It was more
like a state of suspended animation in which my body grew
limp, while my mind remained quasi-alert, listening for the
next reveille.*

*I assumed Skyler wanted to nurse again and he started to.
But then he stopped to emit another opinionated cry, and I
couldn't imagine what it was he wanted now. My husband
rolled over and peered at us, puzzled. Was there anything he
could do? I offered him the part-dazed, part-pleading look he'd
come to know so well. It said: Help me! I don't know what he
wants. Maybe he needs a new diaper. Maybe he's not getting
enough milk. Maybe I ate something too spicy. Maybe the baby
has existential angst. Maybe the baby has gas.*

Off Skyler went in Daddy's arms to the changing table for

a fresh Huggie, but it didn't seem to help. The next thing I heard was the familiar pitter-patter of father feet circling the living room repeatedly while our feisty newborn, with the insistency of a car alarm, attempted to summon the authorities to rescue him from this inept, know-nothing twosome that claimed to be his parents.

I knew my husband thought I should get some sleep while he did his part, but I couldn't sleep when my child was screaming, and besides I now wanted to rescue my valiant spouse who had to get up (as if "getting up" were really some distinguishable dividing line anymore) and get ready for work so soon. So I took the baby from his daddy's arms and settled into a rocking chair by the CD player, where James Taylor proved to have a soporific effect.

With infant breath warming my neck, and the buttery smell of baby scalp in my nostrils, I half-fantasized, half-dreamed. I pictured long, hot showers, uninterrupted slumbers and noonday naps in the sun. I remembered, ever so briefly, what it was like to get into my car and go somewhere on the spur of the moment. I dreamed of lacy nightgowns, the kind without nursing slits cut into the front. Of going to the movies. Of going out to dinner and eating extra spicy curry. At the time, these simple pleasures seemed to me so distant, so forbidden, so forevermore unattainable, that I wept. At the same time I felt guilty for weeping. I loved my baby more than I'd ever imagined. So why wasn't I more reconciled to the sacrifice required?

Later, I was awakened by my husband making breakfast. He was wearing sweatpants and a T-shirt. He wasn't going to work after all. It was Sunday. It was Mother's Day! In front of me was a very large gift-wrapped package which I was startled to see had my name on it, as opposed to our son's. (For six weeks the UPS man had made a daily pilgrimage to our front door bearing satchels of Baby Gap ensembles, the frankincense and myrrh of the 1990s.)

Inside the package was a jogging stroller, the perfect present for someone who was torn between longing to run off

and be free and wanting to stay as tightly tethered as possible
to her tiny, inscrutable, and totally irresistible offspring. . . .

Out of Time

In the late stages of pregnancy, a mother-to-be sometimes wonders aloud about the nitty-gritty specifies of what it will be like to care for her newborn. When will he or she sleep? How often will the child eat? Will he or she cry a lot? But such issues pale beside the advent of her just-around-the-corner childbirth experience, which is often perceived more as an end unto itself than as a moment in time that will change one's life completely.

It is only when birth concludes that we find, often with more surprise than we might have believed possible, that we have crossed a threshold over which there is no returning. With each new baby we must start anew. And as Erik Erikson once said, "It's too bad one must begin with the beginning. We know so little of beginnings."

To start anything at all—a new job, a new semester of school—is difficult. But each of these beginnings is vastly different from the fresh start a mother makes with her fresh-out-of-the-womb baby. As with a beginner in any endeavor, the new mother looks to discover the inherent rhythms and routines of her new circumstances so she can create new habits for herself, and thus get through the days with an increasing degree of ease. But with a brand-new baby there are no set routines, and the only rhythms that can be said to exist conform to a beat far more primal, and unpredictable, than the ticking of our clocks.

The baby wants what he or she wants when he or she wants it. As for the mother, there is no time to reflect on or review her new duties as continual provider. There are breaks in the action, to be sure, for many newborns spend a fair amount of time asleep. But one never knows when the breaks will come, or how long they will last. And somehow or other, they seem to come to an abrupt end just when Mother decides to enter the shower or to catch the first of what she hoped would be forty winks.

Of course, everyone seems to know someone who knows

some other couple who claim their baby slept through the night from Day One and serendipitously seemed to arrange all his waking needs to accommodate Mom and Dad's schedules. Most new mothers say they would give anything to share the charmed fate of such rare and blessed parents. But no one is offering them the option. And, of course, they wouldn't actually trade their particular bundles of joy, quirks and all, for any other baby on the planet.

Indeed, new mothers tend to be so consumed with admiration and adoration for their precious new babies that part of them feels they can endure any hardship, put up with any test, because the reward is so enchanting. But another part of them, the part worn down by so many insistent recurring demands at such frequent and unpatterned intervals, may harbor some supplemental feelings. Like: *Help! My life is over.* Like: *I'll never have a moment to myself again.* Like: *I'll never get out of this bathrobe.*

For it doesn't take long to dawn on the new mother that pregnancy, for all the challenges it presented, was in many aspects a time of luxurious self-preoccupation. Now that time, with all its comparative languor, has vanished all in one irrevocable flash. Suddenly first-time mothers realize that what other women told them, and what they probably tried awfully hard not to hear, turned out to be true: To care for a newborn is to be on constant call. As for "repeater" mothers, they now remember all at once the inevitability of round-the-clock vigilance.

In the time warp that is early postpartum, a mother can hardly help but long for some regularity in her days and nights. And she can't help but mourn the era of her life when she last had ample opportunity to indulge some of her own whims and fancies. Friends and relations may try to remind her, and she may read in the numerous baby-care books she has purchased, that all is not lost, and that at some point—not so far away as she imagines—some semblance of order will be restored to her household, and some degree of liberty (albeit modified for the next eighteen years or so) will be restored to her life. But in her sleep-deprived haze, with her maternal exhilaration tempered by sheer exhaustion, such reassurances may sound like so many muffled and distant foghorns.

Bound inexorably, heart and soul, to her newborn, the new mother is living with her baby outside of time as she usually experiences it. Thus it is hard for her to assimilate the idea that "in time" things will sort themselves out.

If this new mother were living in another type of society, the immediate postpartum days might not feel so overwhelming to her. In many parts of the world, her fatigue might well be mitigated by the fact that it is considered the entitlement of a new mother to forgo all other responsibilities in order to focus solely on her little charge. In India, the Ayurvedic tradition encourages new mothers to stay at home and be pampered for 22 days.[1] In some other nonindustrialized nations, the postpartum pampering period is even longer—often 40 days. Even in some industrialized nations, Mom gets a socially sanctioned break. In England, there are daily visits by health professionals for 14 days after hospital discharge.[2] And in Holland, a trained maternity nurse visits the home of a newborn for 8 to 10 days.[3]

In America, however, many a new mother, tired though she may rightfully be, must not only contend with her newborn solo for many hours a day, but also cope with household chores, answering the phone, greeting the mailman appearing daily with his piles of baby presents, and writing endless thank-you notes. In many cases, she must also keep in some degree of touch with her place of work, which can begin to drive home the fact that juggling a job and a child is likely going to be far more complicated than she ever dreamed. (The challenges of working motherhood are so complex that they deserve an entire book of their own. Fortunately, several good ones are available and can be found in the Suggestions for Further Reading.)

Though many people (especially her well-meaning spouse) may offer assistance and advise her to pace herself, the new mother may find it hard to delegate responsibilities. She may find it somehow embarrassing to say to the world at large what she may long to say, which is: *Slow down, I want to get off!*

She is learning the hard way that newborns have a different relationship to time than just about everyone else in the world.

After their journey in the timeless womb, they have not yet made the transition to linearity. And a new mother does best to surrender herself for a while to living on "baby time" and being interested first and foremost—as is her infant—in moment to moment succor and survival.

The demands of her baby will not go away. Nor should they, of course. The baby is profoundly dependent on his or her mother and must have his or her basic needs met. However, other demands can and should be put in perspective or the mother is apt to go on a woman divided, trying to live by the clock on the wall *and* her baby's internal chronometer. If she insists on doing it all and being the stereotypical Superwoman (curse the person who ever coined the term) she may, ironically enough, delay her departure from the postpartum time tunnel. Too drained to truly stay in tune with her newborn, she'll risk missing the important "This Way Out" signs which her child is probably already posting.

For it is often when the mother begins to decipher her baby's code, to "read" its "language," that her fog begins to lift.

The Learning Curve

During pregnancy a woman mothers on a biological level. All the baby's subsistence needs are met by the placenta, which nourishes the baby and excretes its waste products. Now the mother must meet those basic needs as best she's able, offering breasts, bottles, diapers. She must now mother on a social and emotional level as well. To the baby who was constantly caressed by the walls of her womb and soothed by her heartbeat, she now offers caresses, kisses, and lullabies. But when, and in what fashion, should Mother offer what to baby?

In the beginning, she simply doesn't know. Just as the baby after birth is a stranger in a strange land, so is the baby's mother, who, all at once, is faced with tending a being with whom she can't hold even the simplest of conversations.

There are many questions a mother longs to ask her new child: "Are you sleepy now?" "Do you want more milk?" "Is that diaper dirty?" and the ever-popular *"Why are you crying now?"* But of course the baby is not about to hold forth on these or any other topics. At least not in a way that is immediately comprehensible.

Wanting some sort of guidance, the new mother—especially the first-timer who may feel especially insecure—may look to her baby-care books. While there's nothing wrong with doing some research of this nature, and while it often proves somewhat helpful, she may find that her baby simply hasn't read the same books as she.

A three-hundred-page tome on breast-feeding, read cover to cover, may still fail to enlighten this frustrated mother about the anomalies of her child's nursing habits. A lengthy list of 101 ways to calm a fussy baby may not contain a single suggestion that seems to work consistently for her temperamental tot.

Worse, if she reads avidly and widely, she will find that different child-rearing gurus have diametrically opposed opinions on exactly what ought to be done in a given situation. What is a "mere" mother to think, the mother wonders when even the experts can't agree?

At about this point the new mother will likely begin considering polling her friends and relations as to what they would advise. Often enough, she doesn't even have to start inquiring because advice, in droves, is already on its way. Indeed, it will soon seem that every person who has ever had a child, baby-sat for a child, or seen a child in passing, has a plethora of tips to offer. But these tidbits of wisdom also seem to conflict just as often as not.

Of course, not only rookie mothers may be perplexed by their infants' earliest behaviors. The veteran who already has had a child or two of her own may have thought this time around she would know exactly how to respond to the demands of a tiny baby. The problem is that this tiny baby, like all infants, is a completely unique individual. Brother Bob may have loved bathing in the bathroom sink, where new baby Betsy may scream her tiny lungs out at the prospect. Sister Sue may have stopped crying the second she was put to rock in an infant swing; Brother Sam may go in paroxysms of horror every time that blasted swing is in sight.

Book learning, well-meant advice, firsthand experience with other children—the new mother quickly comes to understand that all of it only goes so far. Waxing nostalgic for what she now recalls as the "simplicity" of pregnancy, she must face the fact that she is near the base of a learning curve, a curve which will ascend steeply before beginning to level off for a spell.

Over the next weeks, some of her best tools for understanding her baby will be her powers of observation and her willingness to partake in some trial and error. The more she is able to temporarily defer or delegate other tasks (the phone call from the office, the thank-you correspondence) to study her baby, the more quickly she'll become *the* definitive expert on her child.

Intuition certainly plays a role in picking up on the needs of one's infant. And it's true that, on occasion, a new mother will have a pretty good hunch about how to deal with a baby's desire without consciously understanding where she got her insight. But expecting total telepathy is unrealistic and self-defeating. Learning to understand one's baby is, for the most part, an *acquired* skill.

With a bit of patience, even the most baffled new mother will soon enough come to know, by listening to the timbre and rhythm of her baby's cry, and watching the subtle expressions on her face, when she's tired or hungry, or when she's about to dirty her diaper.

"When I first brought my daughter home," recalled first-time mother 27-year-old Jessica, "I felt so inadequate because I'd heard that a mother would know what her child's cries were trying to communicate. At first they all sounded completely alike to me. I had no idea what she wanted. Then I began to realize there *were* differences. By the time she was a couple of months old, for example, I knew that the whiny cry that sounded like a lawn mower that couldn't quite kick into gear meant she was sleepy. So then instead of picking her up and carrying her around when I heard that cry— which usually made her cry harder—I learned that what she actually wanted was to be put down. I'd rub her back for a minute, and she'd be off to dreamland. I was so proud I understood her. It was like finding the Rosetta stone."

With enough perseverance, trying a little of this and a little of that, a new mother will soon come to understand what stimulates her baby and what soothes him:

"My son cried so loud and hard every night for the first couple of months of his life," said 33-year-old Joanna of her second child, "that even our dog would hide under the bed in distress. At first I tried everything his older brother seemed to like when he was a baby. I bounced him on my knee, I put him in a baby carrier. Forget it. I tried a baby swing. No way. So then I tried singing every lullaby I could think of, and finally something clicked. Don't ask me why, but every time I sang *Frère Jacques*—in French, mind you, not English—he would get this blissful look on this face and calm down instantly. What can I say? Maybe he was French in a past life. I don't know. I just stumbled across this little trick, but it always worked like a charm.

Amazingly enough, before long a mother will be able to do what her baby "tells" her without really stopping to think about it. She will be able to instruct others with some degree of assurance and authority.

"The first day I spent alone at home with my daughter Kaitlin, I had the eeriest feeling," recalled 30-year-old Andrea, a first-time mother. "I remember sitting in my living room, holding her, staring at her perfect face and thinking, *'So, I wonder when the mother is coming.'* I just felt so clueless. I couldn't imagine myself in that role. A few months later I went back to work part-time and I found myself typing out eight pages of instructions for the baby-sitter. I wrote: *When Kaitie does such and such, she means so-and-so. When it's bath time, she likes this. When it's nap time, she likes that.* I knew I had actually grown into the role of mother—that I was the person who was 'coming' all along."

It almost goes without saying that as you get a firmer handle on what your baby expects of you and how the baby expresses himself or herself, you will feel more in control. With an increase in the sense of control, comes a decrease in the overwhelming sense of confusion and fatigue many new mothers experience. Hence a decrease in stress. Though the job of mothering still requires tremendous stamina, and always will, it's likely your anxiety will be lessened once you have a yardstick by which to measure what's "normal" for your baby.

When it comes to learning about babies, babies themselves are the greatest teachers. It's as if they come preprogrammed to release their mothers' potential. Naturally, there will be glitches along the way. And it's not at all unusual to feel that mother-hood is one of those two-steps-forward, one-step-back proc-esses. That is in fact its essence. And never more so than during the transitional time of the first few months.

All transitions are disconcerting. All are frustrating. All are complicated. If you sometimes wonder during the first months you spend with your baby if you'll ever get the hang of it, you are having very typical feelings indeed.

But often new mothers want to know if their particular feel-ings and frustrations fall within the realm of "routine" postpar-tum adjustments, or whether they've somehow crossed a line. Having heard the term "postpartum depression" (or PPD) you may at some point wonder if you have it. And if you think you do have it, what can you do about it?

Shades of Blue

Depression of any sort is believed to have several possible root causes. It can be a direct result of feeling helpless. It can be cre-ated when feelings of anger are turned inward, directed against the self instead of at someone else. It can be at least partially biochemically based, a result of an "imbalance" of sorts in the brain. In any case, it is easy to see why the mother of a new baby might be predisposed toward feeling, to one degree or another, depressed.

Biochemical readjustments may well influence a new moth-er's mood as the hormonal balance that was achieved during pregnancy unwinds. But, once again, the entire key does not lie in the endocrine system. Adoptive mothers have certainly been known to become depressed once their babies arrive, though they have not been through the physical childbirth process.

As for the helplessness factor, as we've already seen, it's only natural to feel helpless in the early phases of caring for a being so insistent on getting what it needs, and yet so hard to make sense of. As for anger, whether one would like to believe this or not, it's perfectly natural to get angry when first trying to cope with all the demands of mothering a newborn. Even D. W. Winnicott, the pediatrician and psychoanalyst so well known for his empathic perspective on children, compiled a rather lengthy list of reasons why mothers might get mad at their babies. Among the many reasons he enumerated: "The baby is an interference with her private life." "The baby at first must dominate." And: "After an awful morning with him she goes out, and he smiles at a stranger, who says, 'Isn't he sweet?' "[4]

Typically, the mother doesn't vent her anger *at* her baby, deeming this an unacceptable option. But beyond that, she may even be ashamed to express her frustrations to others, such as her spouse or friends, because she fears that her being mad might come off as being "bad." Here, alas, we have optimum conditions for anger turning against the self. For the psychic energy attached to an emotion must do something, go somewhere. When we won't let it out somehow, it simply has no place else to go but inward.

In addition to all these potentially predisposing factors to depression, the new mother has others. For one thing, she may feel—and in fact truly be—isolated. Once the initial parade of baby-ogling visitors has subsided, and once Dad goes back to work, she may face long days at home alone with her baby who, for all his or her charms, is not about to engage with her in a chat about the morning headlines or challenge her to a good game of Scrabble.

For another thing, a new mother's marriage may not offer quite the degree of predictable solace it did before. The new baby in the house means husband and wife need to try new roles on for size, rearrange their schedules, renegotiate their respective responsibilities. More often than not, there may be a few bumps on the road to a redefined relationship.

Many new mothers feel "abandoned" by their husbands.

"A week after our son was born," recalled 33-year-old Claudia, "my husband had to go back to work. It was a critical time in his business year and I knew he really had no choice. I knew he couldn't stay home indefinitely and believed him when he said he'd rather be with us. Nevertheless I wept inconsolably every time he called during the day to say hello. I'd say, 'How can you do this to me. How can you leave me like this?' "

"My husband was just as helpful as he could be," said 28-year-old Gail, "but because I was nursing, there was obviously one thing I was entirely responsible for. At those midnight and 2 A.M. and 4 A.M. feedings, I remember feeling like the loneliest person in the world. Sometimes I felt so resentful. It may sound irrational, but I would be fuming because he didn't have mammary glands."

And many fear they now play "second fiddle" in their partners' affections.

"You know it may sound like a small thing," said 30-year-old Faith, "but before the baby was born, my husband and I had this silly little ritual way of greeting each other when we got home from work. We'd just kind of hum and slow dance around the kitchen for a minute.

"After our daughter was born, my husband would come in, pick her up and dance before I even got a kiss. Part of me loved to see him be such a good dad. But part of me was really hurt, like I had been cast aside."

Also, as during pregnancy itself, the new mother may reexperience some unresolved feelings of sadness emanating from her own early infancy, especially if her circumstances were marked by some significant deprivation. And she may identify with her own baby to such an extent that she has difficulty separating out when the baby's upset versus when she's upset.

Lingering regrets about a disappointing or traumatic birth

experience can also be a contributing factor to depression, as may unrealistically high expectations about what mothering would actually be like.

Additionally, any woman who has had an unwanted pregnancy, previous depressive episodes, a major significant loss or move or other life change in the past two years may also be predisposed to postnatal feelings of depression. *But none of these extenuating circumstances need exist for postpartum depression to occur.* Indeed anyone with a new baby at home, no matter what her age, economic class, or life-style (and no matter whether she's experienced postpartum depression with past births or not) may potentially fall into a depressed state.

Given all this, it's interesting that the number of new mothers who merit an official diagnosis of postpartum depression is estimated to be only around 20 percent. But psychological diagnosis is tricky business, often more of a judgment call than a precise science. Remember, at least four out of five mothers are estimated to have the "baby blues" shortly after birth. And the line between where "blues" ends and "depression" begins is, in reality, quite fuzzy.

Consider some criteria said to be indicative of a case of baby blues: anxiety, irritability, low energy, lack of confidence, worry. Now consider some of the symptoms typically said to indicate postpartum depression: anxiety and irritability (that familiar combination), exhaustion (as in lack of energy, only presumably more extreme), feelings of inadequacy (as in lack of confidence, only presumably more pronounced), overconcern for baby (as in worry, only presumably more intense).

The lists go on, both including various degrees of nervousness, guilt, disorientation, hypersensitivity, mood swings, crying bouts, appetite and sleep disturbances. Certainly there are some symptoms that are said to fall more clearly under the purview of postpartum depression per se, for example physical sensations such as heart palpitations and hyperventilation, and behavioral reactions such as panic attacks, new phobias, and even hallucinations. But certainly not all sufferers of postpartum depression evidence these latter manifestations.

Ironically, this diagnostic vagueness can itself be a source of stress to any new mother who may attempt to look up her plight in a book, wanting to know, *Where do I fit in?* But rather than getting bogged down with terminology, or seeking labels and categories to pigeonhole themselves, women would do best to conceive of postpartum depression as existing on a continuum, with symptoms ranging from mild to moderate to severe. The ultimate rule of thumb for any woman who feels her adjustment to motherhood is a source of despondency: *Do not suffer silently, reach out and get help without hesitation.*

Professional help is one possible route. A new mother may find that simply engaging in some short-term psychotherapy with a therapist familiar with postpartum issues is enough to work through the aspects of adjustment to parenthood she finds most daunting. She may even elect to have her husband participate in some of the therapy sessions so that they can discuss their shifting relationship and so that Dad can have a chance to discuss any depression he himself may be experiencing. (Not surprisingly, new fathers are not immune from PPD.)

On occasion, a professional may deem a case of PPD so serious that medication is considered. While this might prove beneficial in severe cases, medication should only be prescribed by a doctor who is extremely knowledgeable about postpartum depression. If not, the mother risks taking a long ride of a chemical merry-go-round. (If she is breast-feeding, for example, she will have to stop doing so once she's medicated, and the very act of ceasing nursing will itself alter her hormonal balance yet again.)

Apart from enlisting professional help, many women find that support groups are an invaluable tool for coping with the feelings associated with PPD. Simply getting together with other new mothers and sharing fears and frustrations is often experienced as emerging from darkness into light. Because now the secret is out. There are countless others out there who have emotions like hers! It is wonderful for any new mother to know that she is not the only one who sometimes feels stressed or lonely or mad or frightened, or who is experiencing the "culture shock" of adapting to the many unknowns her new baby has introduced into her household.

It is wonderful too for her to be given the opportunity to

discover that feeling depressed or angry or overwhelmed or anything else does not make her less of a "good mother." It's what
one *does* with feelings that is critical. To openly air them with
people who can empathize, as opposed to bottling them up
where they can cause internal havoc, is to put them to constructive use.

Out of the Woods

It would be wrong to say that talking things out is a panacea for
the new mother, who will have new challenges to rise to for
quite some time to come. But it helps enormously. And, whether
done on a formal or informal basis, it is something that many
may find an invaluable tool for negotiating the entire first postpartum year.

One of the prevalent myths of postpartum recovery is that it
ends in six weeks or so, and that at this juncture a woman is
again her former self in every way. This widespread misunder-
standing is based on the fact that doctors say it takes approxi-
mately six weeks for the uterus to return to pre-pregnancy size.
But this development does not necessarily mean other postpartum symptoms, both physical and psychological, will abruptly
subside.

As new mothers themselves have long known, and as a recent extensive University of Minnesota study has proven for the
record, physical symptoms and syndromes such as digestive
problems, breast discomfort, discomfort during intercourse,
poor appetite, acne, increased perspiring, numbness and tingling
of the hands, hot flashes, respiratory ailments, and, of course,
fatigue often persist for a new mother well into her baby's first
year of life.[5] The emotional ramifications of mothering an infant—from feeling anxious and overwhelmed to frustrated to
guilty to depressed to generally conflicted—are also wont to persist, albeit in varying degrees at various times, well into the first
year. Why wouldn't they?

For the majority of its premier year of life, and especially in
the first several months, a baby's existence revolves around its

mother. For her part, the mother makes meeting her baby's needs an exceedingly high priority, even when that means making difficult sacrifices, and making them repeatedly. Not to have at least occasional mixed feelings about this continuing maternal requirement and all it entails is not to be human. And to pretend not to have them is counterproductive.

Of course, babies won't always need their mothers as intently as they do at the very start. Indeed, by the time they are only four or five months of age they embark on a journey of separation and individuation that child development researcher Margaret Mahler has referred to as "hatching." To begin, the baby molds himself or herself less to the mother's body and gazes beyond her periphery. The child becomes more active and slides down from her lap, flirting with the world beyond.

By nine or ten months, in a period Mahler calls "the psychological birth," the baby becomes enamored with the wide world and all it contains. Though Mother still takes precedence over other people and external objects, she has some stiff competition. The child is readying himself or herself for greater independence. And it's believed to be no coincidence that when the baby starts to walk, its first steps tend to be in a direction away from its mother.[6]

But now the mother has something else to have mixed feelings about. Her needy little one's not so needy or so little anymore. And though there are years of togetherness ahead, the writing is already on the wall: Someday (sigh) he'll be grown up and gone away.

No one ever said mothering a new baby would be easy. (At least no female who has reproduced has ever said it.) Every woman must come to terms with it in her own way and *in her own time*. Having physical or emotional expectations of oneself based on any supposedly "average" postpartum time frame is a mistake.

You know when you feel okay and when something is troubling you. No matter how many weeks or months have elapsed since your baby's birth, if you feel you're not out of the woods, find some fellow travelers, and perhaps an experienced guide as well. With their assistance, you can discover a path that is navigable for you, for your baby, for your family.

❖ A NEW MOTHER'S PRIVILEGES AND PREROGATIVES

Ask for help. You'll need it! Many of us have been conditioned to view independence as a lofty goal. When you're a new mother, allowing yourself to ask for help is an even higher goal to aspire to. With a new baby (and any baby is someone new, even if you have had others) you are a novice. Your work is cut out for you in that you have to figure out who this baby is and what he or she wants. No matter how accomplished you may be in the outside world, this particular achievement must be tackled slowly and carefully. While you attend to it as a primary duty, enlist the assistance of your spouse, your parents, your neighbors, and your friends.

If relying on family and friends is not possible (perhaps you've moved to a new community of late and lack this sort of support system; or perhaps you feel there is too much emotional baggage involved in counting on, say, your mother or mother-in-law), seriously consider obtaining professional help. Do as much as your budget can possibly accommodate. Hire someone to clean your house. Send the laundry out. Order phone food. Investigate (while you're still pregnant, if possible) some of the new services which are springing up around the country which train and provide postpartum helpers (sometimes referred to as *doulas*). They will do anything from assisting with newborn care to housekeeping to shopping to sending out birth announcements. (See the Resources Section at the end of his book for help in locating such helpers.)

Take charge of the traffic flow. Watch out for social isolation but also watch out for being inundated early on with visitors who wish to see your family's newest member. I know a woman who, after her baby's birth, hung a sign on her door which she got from her midwife. It said: *Baby so-and-so was born at such and such a time/ Mom and baby are fine/ Please limit your stay as both need to rest/ If while you're here, you can throw in a load of wash, clear dishes, or fix a meal, the whole family would appreciate it.* As she explained, this sort of communication "plants the seed of awareness in visitors that a post-birth visit is not about just admiring baby, but supporting a whole family."

Listen to your body, and set only realistic goals. After birth, it is important to rest as much as is humanly possible under the circumstances. It is a big mistake to try to resume certain arduous activities—from vigorous exercise to housecleaning to writing legal briefs on deadline—too soon. Heed your body's signals. If your bleeding gets heavier when you vacuum the house, *stop vacuuming.* If you feel uncomfortable doing fifty sit-ups or power walking on a treadmill, hold off for the time being and begin again more gradually. If you feel like you're going to hyperventilate every time the office calls, defer or at least limit those calls. You have the rest of your life to push papers, push a broom, or climb a Stairmaster. Postnatal time is a time to mother and be mothered. Eat well. Get a massage. Take responsibility for your physical well-being, or ultimately you and your baby, not to mention everyone else in the household, will be shortchanged.

As when pregnant, take advice with a large dose of salt. Some people say bathe babies this way; some say bathe them that way. Some say, "Feed them on a schedule." Some say, "Feed them on demand." Some say, "Let them cry a few nights and then they'll sleep through." Some say, "That's cruel," or "That never works." Some say, "Don't talk baby talk to them." Some say, "Echo whatever they do." Which way is the right way for you and your baby? Ultimately, only you can decide, based on your needs and the needs your baby communicates to you. If you end up doing things differently than your mother did, or your friends and colleagues do, so be it. Remember, with a new baby, trial and error is the name of the game.

Forget about being perfect, or even approaching it. Mothers of newborns who expect never to make mistakes (either because they're idealistic first-timers or because they're veteran moms who assume prior experience will enable them to put in a flawless performance this time around) are in for a rude awakening. No mother, neither you nor anyone else, can meet all of her baby's needs perfectly all the time, no matter how legitimate those needs may be. Try not to obsess on your occasional "slip-ups." They're not only forgivable, they're necessary for your child's healthy development. After all, imagine the child who grows up having his or her every wish instantly gratified every minute of the day and night. The child would be unable to tolerate frustration (of which life, alas, is full), unable to develop patience or self-reliance or even a sense of humor. It's not a pretty picture. So be grateful you're not able to render it.

Cultivate mutually supportive relationships with other mothers. New mothers are everywhere. You'll find them on your block, at the park playground, at church, and at work (if and when you return to work). Even if you don't feel you have a postpartum depression issue to resolve, seek these women out. Share information, share a gripe session, share a laugh. If at all possible, arrange to get together on a regular basis (with babies in tow if you like). Such networking has countless benefits, both practical and psychical. Just when you begin to think your child is the most unusual and unpredictable creature ever to be born of womankind, you'll find out from your compatriots that there are indeed other babies who: a) never fall asleep until David Letterman is off the air; b) only spit up on dry-cleanables; c) are able to spread Zweibach paste on an entire sofa in the time it takes you to answer the doorbell; or d) all of the above. Something about this usually makes one feel better.

Keep Dad in the loop. No matter how much you and your spouse planned how things would be after the birth, whether in terms of how you'd share baby duty or how you'd keep your relationship spontaneous and romantic, things may veer off onto a different course once your baby actually arrives. As you know, some women feel somewhat "deserted" by their husbands during the postpartum period. If you have such feelings, they should be brought up with your partner in a way he can tolerate, so he can understand your view without getting defensive. But, in addition, don't neglect to examine what role you may be playing in any marital discord.

For example, you may find yourself so glued to your infant that Dad hardly has a chance to do his share. Or you may find you are so consumed with motherhood that you tend to back-burner your marriage without even realizing it. Although it is vital that you spend a great deal of time tuning in to your baby, do not tune your partner out. In the long run, all of you will be happier if you encourage your baby's father to bond with his child as much as possible.

Like all couples with new babies at home, you two will undoubtedly have a lot to work through. All of you, including your baby, will be much stronger if your marital bond remains strong. So please see the Suggestions for Further Reading for sources to consult on the vast topic of how parenthood impacts a marriage.

Do your child a favor—accept yourself and your emotions. Just as mothers tune in to their babies, babies tune in to their mothers. Your infant is very sensitive to what's going on with you. If you find yourself pressing down feelings such as sadness, anger, or anxiety in an attempt to shield your baby, know that it simply will not work. Unacknowledged feelings only intensify. And like a small but absorbent sponge, your baby can potentially soak up the overflow. In this way, an infant may be psychologically "programmed" to grow up acting out all the feelings you won't allow yourself to claim as your own.

If you can express all your feelings, you will find that your child will grow up retaining the ability to express all of his or hers—and they will be truly his or hers, genuine expressions of his or her inner self. So, for your child's sake as well as your own, find appropriate outlets for your emotions. (But do not judge yourself harshly for the occasional outburst, for it's hard to be "appropriate" all the time.)

The bottom line is that if you can't accept yourself, you can't really accept your child. What a sorrow that would be. For accepting one another—on good days and bad, with ups, downs, and in-betweens, with shortcomings and crowning glories—is what love is really all about.

EPILOGUE

Happy Birthday to Us

Yesterday I wrote the final paragraphs of the final chapter of this book. Tomorrow, incredibly, is my son's first birthday. This morning I ran around town hunting down crepe paper streamers and helium balloons. I gathered up food and drink for tomorrow's party guests. I ordered an ice-cream cake and bought a big "1" candle to place on top. I called my parents, who were leaving for the Fort Lauderdale airport to come join the festivities, to remind them that March in the Northeast is still overcoat weather. I wondered if I had forgotten anything and concluded that I probably had, and would just have to wing it at some point. I've become rather adept at winging it this past year, as has my husband, because no day has been quite like the day before.

My son hasn't really seemed to have noticed our improvisations, though, or if he has he hasn't seemed to mind. I suppose he realizes on some level that his parents are raw but eager and educable. And he's surviving our gradual enlightenment rather nicely.

I'm proud to report that Skyler has managed, in his first twelve months of life, to put on sixteen pounds, shoot up nine inches, cut eight teeth, and grow an absolutely bewildering head full of thick, shiny, light brown hair. He's an enthusiastic connoisseur of crackers, yogurt, and bananas, a master of peeka-

boo, and an ace at emptying out Daddy's dresser drawers and Mama's lower file cabinets. An early walker, he routinely astonishes the neighbors by toddling down our driveway, waving, and saying "hi" in twelve-month-old lingo ("Da-Da!"). They tell him what a big boy he is, and lately, aware that his birthday was just around the bend, they have been asking me, "Didn't the year go fast?"

Well, yes. And no. In a way it does seem like yesterday that our baby was so weensy we could strap him across our chests and take a stroll down to the local duck pond barely noticing the extra weight we were carrying. But to be honest there were certain days (generally the ones following almost totally sleepless nights) which seemed to stretch on interminably. I'd spend those dazed days mopping up projectile rice cereal, calculating whether or not we had enough diapers to postpone a trip to the A&P, and wishing in vain that I had enough residual brain cells to attempt something more complicated like, say, paying the gas bill. In all, I wouldn't say the year passed in a blink, but I'm sure the older Sky gets, the more it will seem so.

The way we remember is so subjective. Many things compress, many things fade. In a way, I've kept the memories of my pregnancy unusually vivid by immersing myself in this project. Friends who were pregnant at the same time as I already sense their recollections receding. I suppose it will not be long before that brilliant time in my life glows dimmer and dimmer and is recalled more simply and concisely: I conceived, I grew large, I felt very emotional, I had a baby, and now I have a few good stories to pass along.

That compression is as it should be, I suppose. Pregnancy is intense and immediate. It is urgent business. But life careens along, and one of the things pregnancy instructs us in is that things must be savored in the moment. It intructs us in other matters as well. Whether we want it to or not it teaches us a thing or two about tolerance, about responsibility, about discipline, about courage. It teaches us about power—our own and that of forces greater than any one of us. It alerts us to our own deepest longings and deepest doubts. It gives us a shot at the brass ring of hope and faith. And if we give it half a chance, it strengthens each of us in the particular ways we need to be strengthened.

So what if the precise memories tend to pale? We are forever altered, and when we need to access the self-knowledge with which pregnancy endowed us, I believe we do so more or less instinctively. The information of pregnancy is now part of our mothering database.

But enough philosophizing. Even as I speak, the birthday boy is calling to me from down the hall. Dad's been engaging him in a favorite pastime, bang-the-spatula-on-the-salad-spinner. But he's on the prowl for Mama now and as soon as he finds me he'll want to evict me from my desk chair so he can sit in it and spin. And who can blame him? I'd like to spin a bit myself, get a little goofy, clang a pot against a pan, jump up and down and squeal in sheer delight. Hey, I deserve it. And so will you. Because after all: We conceived, we grew large, we felt very emotional, we had our babies, and now we have a few good stories to pass along.

ENDNOTES

CHAPTER 1

1. Jacques Gélis, *History of Childbirth* (Boston: Northeastern University Press, 1991), p. 47.

CHAPTER 2

1. Diane Ackerman, *A Natural History of the Senses* (New York: Random House, 1990), pp. 149–150.
2. Gélis, op. cit. p. 56.
3. *U.S. News & World Report* (July 29, 1992), p. 61.
4. *The New York Times* (October 25, 1992), Section 9, p. 1.
5. Annick LeGuérer, *Scent: The Mysterious and Essential Powers of Smell* (New York: Turtle Bay Books, 1992), p. 24.
6. Ibid., as quoted on p. 157.
7. Jean-Jacques Rousseau, *Ouevres complètes*, Vol. III (Paris: Gallimard, 1969), p. 140.
8. Judith Goldsmith, *Childbirth Wisdom* (Brookline, Mass.: East West Health Books, 1990), p. 13.
9. Gélis, op. cit. p. 83.
10. *U.S. News & World Report*, op. cit.
11. *Mothering* (Winter 1984), p. 55.
12. Gélis, op. cit. pp. 69–73.

CHAPTER 3

1. Perri Klass, "Bearing a Child in Medical School," *The New York Times Magazine* (November 11, 1984), pp. 124–125.

2. *The Pregnant Patient's Responsibilities* (Minneapolis: International Childbirth Education Association, Inc.)

3. Robbie E. Davis-Floyd, *Birth as an American Rite of Passage* (Berkeley and Los Angeles: University of California Press, 1992), p. 299. (This reference is the source only of the statistics in the footnoted passage.)

4. Sheila Kitzinger, *Mothering* (Spring, 1990), p. 63.

5. Melvin Konner, M.D., *Becoming a Doctor* (New York: Viking, 1987), p. 223.

6. Joseph B. DeLee, *The Principles and Practice of Obstetrics* (Philadelphia: W. B. Saunders, 1940), as cited in Jessica Mitford's *The American Way of Birth* (New York: Dutton, 1992), p. 53.

7. Klass, op. cit. p. 125.

8. *Mothering* (Spring, 1993), p. 81.

CHAPTER 4

1. Libby Lee and Arthur D. Colman, *Pregnancy: The Psychological Experience* (New York: The Seabury Press, 1971), p. 76.

2. *Vanity Fair* (August, 1992), p. 118.

3. Gélis, op. cit. p. 67.

4. Carol Tavris, *The Mismeasure of Woman* (New York: Simon & Schuster, 1992), p. 120.

5. Gélis, op. cit. p. 82.

CHAPTER 5

1. *The New Yorker* (August 11, 1980), p. 21.

2. Marc McCutcheon, *The Compass in Your Nose* (Los Angeles: Jeremy P. Tarcher, Inc., 1989), p. 84.

3. Gélis, op. cit. p. 51.

4. Thomas Verny, M.D., & Pamela Weintraub, *Nurturing the Unborn Child* (New York: Delacorte Press, 1991), pp. 104–105.

5. Ibid., p. xxiii.

6. Ibid., p. xxv.

CHAPTER 6

1. Goldsmith, op. cit. pp. 11–13.

2. Ibid.

3. Jessica Mitford, *The American Way of Birth* (New York: Dutton, 1992), p. 71.

4. Anne Hooper, *The Ultimate Sex Book: A Therapist's Guide to Sexual Fulfillment* (London: Dorling Kindersley, 1992), p. 130.

5. Ibid.

CHAPTER 7

1. Deborah Tannen, *The New York Times Magazine* (June 20, 1993), p. 18.

2. *The Wall Street Journal* (May 19, 1993), p. B1.

3. Caroline Whitbeck, "Theories of Sex Difference," *The Philosophical Forum* (1973, Vol. 5), pp. 1–2.

4. Barbara Rothman, *Recreating Motherhood* (New York: Norton, 1989), p. 248.

5. Ibid.

6. Davis-Floyd, op. cit. p. 25.

CHAPTER 8

1. Klass, op. cit. pp. 123–124.

2. Ibid.

3. S. M. Tobin, "Emotional Depression During Pregnancy," *Obstetrics and Gynecology* Vol. 10 (1957), p. 677.

4. Gayle Peterson, *Birthing Normally* (Berkeley: Shadow and Light, 1981), p. 195.

CHAPTER 9

1. *Newsweek* (June 28, 1993), p. 6.

2. Livingston F. Jones, *A Study of the Tlingets of Alaska* (New York: Fleming H. Revell, 1914) (as quoted in Goldsmith's *Childbirth Wisdom*, p. 23).

3. Konner, op. cit. p. 211.

4. Ibid., p. 212.

5. Susan McCutcheon-Rosegg, with Peter Rosegg, *Natural Childbirth the Bradley Way* (New York: Plume, 1984), p. 115–116.

6. Davis-Floyd, op. cit. p. 155.

7. Marshall H. Klaus, M.D.; John H. Kennell, M.D.; and Phyllis H. Klaus, M.Ed., C.S.W., *Mothering the Mother* (Reading, Mass: Addison-Wesley, 1993), p. 118.

CHAPTER 10

1. Robin Lim, *After the Baby's Birth . . . A Woman's Way to Wellness* (Berkeley, CA: Celestial Arts, 1991), p. 7.

2. Klaus, et. al., op. cit. p. 117.

3. *Mothering* (Spring, 1993), p. 81.

4. D. W. Winnicott, *Through Paediatrics to Psycho-Analysis* (New York: Basic Books, 1958), p. 201.

5. *Parents* (August, 1993), p. 64.

6. Margaret S. Mahler, Fred Pine, and Anni Bergman, *The Psychological Birth of the Human Infant* (Basic Books: New York, 1975), p. 73.

RESOURCE LIST

For General Information on All Aspects of Childbirth:

AMERICAN COLLEGE OF NURSE MIDWIVES (ACNM)
1522 K St. NW, Suite 1000
Washington, DC 20005
(202) 289-0171

AMERICAN COLLEGE OF OBSTETRICIANS AND GYNECOLOGISTS
409 12 St. NW
Washington, DC 20024
(202) 638-5577

INTERNATIONAL ASSOCIATION OF PARENTS AND PROFESSIONALS FOR SAFE
    ALTERNATIVES IN CHILDBIRTH (NAPSAC)
Route 1, Box 646
Marble Hill, MO 63764
(314) 238-2010

INTERNATIONAL CHILDBIRTH EDUCATION ASSOCIATION, INC. (ICEA)
P.O. Box 20048
Minneapolis, MN 55420
(612) 854-8660

For Labor and/or Postpartum Information and Support:

DOULAS OF NORTH AMERICA (DONA)
1100 23rd Ave. E.
Seattle, WA 98112
FAX: (206) 325-0472

NATIONAL ASSOCIATION OF CHILDBIRTH ASSISTANTS (NACA)
219 Meridian Ave.
San Jose, CA 95126
(408) 225-9167

NATIONAL ASSOCIATION OF POSTPARTUM CARE SERVICES (NAPCS)
8910 29th Place SW
Edmonds, WA 98206

For Postpartum Depression Support Groups:

DEPRESSION AFTER DELIVERY
P.O. Box 1282
Morrisville, PA 19067
(215) 295-3994
(800) 944-4773

For Breast-feeding Information and Support:

INTERNATIONAL LACTATION CONSULTANT ASSOCIATION
P.O. Box 4031
University of Virginia Station
Charlottesville, VA 22903

LA LECHE LEAGUE INTERNATIONAL
9615 Minneapolis Ave.
Franklin Park, IL 60131
1-800-LA-LECHE

SUGGESTIONS FOR FURTHER READING

ABOUT CHILDBIRTH AND FINDING A PRACTITIONER:

Birth As an American Rite of Passage by Robbie E. Davis-Floyd (University of California Press, 1992)

The Birth Book by William Sears, M.D., and Martha Sears, R.N. (Little Brown, 1994)

Birthing Normally: A Personal Growth Approach to Childbirth by Gayle Peterson (Shadow and Light, Second Edition 1984)

The Birth Partner: Everything You Need to Know to Help a Woman Through Childbirth by Penny Simkin (The Harvard Common Press, 1989)

The Midwife's Pregnancy and Childbirth Book: Having Your Baby Your Way by Marion McCartney, CNM, and Antonia van der Meer (Harper Perennial, 1991)

Mothering the Mother: How a Doula Can Help You Have a Shorter, Easier, and Healthier Birth by Marshall H. Klauss, M.D.; John H. Kennell, M.D.; and Phyllis H. Klaus, M.Ed., C.S.W. (Addison-Wesley, 1993)

Natural Childbirth the Bradley Way by Susan McCutcheon-Rosegg with Peter Rosegg (Plume, 1984) Note: Even for those not necessarily interested in the Bradley Method per se, this book contains such worthy chapters as "The Emotional Map of Labor."

Sense and Sensibility in Childbirth: A Guide to Supportive Obstetrical Care by Judith Herzfeld, Ph.D. (Norton, 1985)

EXERCISE, YOGA, AND BEAUTY:

The Complete Pregnancy Exercise Program by Diana Simkin (Plume, 1980)

Essential Exercises for the Childbearing Year by Elizabeth Nobel (Houghton Mifflin, 1988)
The Pregnant Woman's Beauty Book by Gloria Natale (Morrow, 1980)
A Year of Beauty and Exercise for Pregnancy by Jidi Mahon (Lippincott & Crowell, 1980)
Yoga for Pregnancy: Safe and Gentle Stretches by Sandra Jordan (St. Martin's, 1987)

PRENATAL "COMMUNICATION":

Nurturing the Unborn Child by Thomas Verny, M.D., & Pamela Weintraub (Delacorte Press, 1991)

BREAST-FEEDING:

Keys to Breastfeeding by William Sears, M.D., and Martha Sears, R.N. (Barron's, 1991)
The Womanly Art of Breastfeeding (5th revised edition) by La Leche League International (Plume, 1991)

POSTPARTUM AND NEW MOTHER ISSUES:

After the Baby's Birth . . . A Woman's Way to Wellness by Robin Lim (Celestial Arts, 1991)
Mother Care by Lyn Delli Quadri and Kati Breckenridge (Tarcher, 1978)
Motherhood: What It Does to Your Mind by Jane Price (Pandora Press, 1988)
The Myth of the Bad Mother: Parenting Without Guilt by Jane Swigart, Ph.D. (Avon, 1991)

SEX AND MARRIAGE:

Childbirth and Marriage: The Transition to Parenthood by Tracy Hotcher (Avon, 1988)
Making Love During Pregnancy by Elizabeth Bing and Libby Colman (Bantam, 1977)
When Partners Become Parents: The Big Life Change for Couples by Carolyn P. Cowan (Basic Books, 1993)

FOR WORKING MOTHERS:

Everything a Working Mother Needs to Know by Anne C. Weisberg and Carol A. Buckler (Main Street/Doubleday, 1994)

How to Have a Child and Keep Your Job by Jane Price (St. Martin's, 1979)

Managing Your Maternity Leave by Meg Wheatley and Marcie Schorr (Houghton Mifflin, 1983)

My Mother Worked and I Turned Out Okay by Katherine Goldman (Villard, 1993)

Of Cradles and Careers: A Guide to Reshaping Your Job to Include a Baby in Your Life by Kaye Lowman (La Leche League International, 1984)

The Preschool Years by Ellen Galinsky and Judy David (Ballantine, 1993) Note: includes review of research on known effects of maternal employment.

The Working Mother's Baby Planner by Marla Schram Scwartz (Prentice Hall, 1993) Note: a handy workbook to have while you're still pregnant.

Keys to Choosing Child Care by Stevanne Auerbach (Barron's, 1991)

FOR FATHERS:

Earth Father, Sky Father: The Changing Concept of Fathering by Arthur and Libby Colman (Prentice Hall, 1981)

The Father Book by Rae Grad (Acropolis, 1982)

Keys to Becoming a Father by William Sears, M.D. (Barron's, 1991)

Pregnant Fathers by Jack Heinowitz (Spectrum, 1982)